The Postpartum Book for Partners

A Comprehensive Look at the Fourth Trimester, Balancing Becoming a New Parent and Supporting Your Partner Without Forgetting Yourself

Theresa Charles

Table of Contents

Introduction

Becoming a parent can feel scary for everyone involved. There are guidebooks for pregnancy, labor, and birth, which give you an idea of what to expect, but you never know what it will be like until you actually experience it. And then, you're left with a newborn and a faint hope that things will go okay. It's alarming how the guidance for new parents dries up once their baby is born—when you actually need the most help! Some people are lucky and have trusted family and friends to help them in those first few weeks of their baby's life, but that type of advice can often seem overbearing. Once someone starts giving you tips, it can be hard to get them to stop, and an awkward conversation is the last thing you need when you're already struggling to navigate your new life. And those who don't have trustworthy people helping them through this sleep-deprived journey might have even more uncertainty than they know how to handle.

With that in mind, I wanted to put my experience to good use. After the birth of my first child, I felt so alone and unsupported. I eventually found a few postpartum resources for mothers, but realized my husband was left in the dark. He read the same information I did, but it mostly referred to my body, health, and healing. There weren't many resources out there for first-time dads. We navigated those waters together, helping each other through, but it was taxing for both of us. I knew I didn't want anyone else to go through that uncertain experience while also striving to become a great parent. First-time dads are going through a major life change, and having a handy guide is a great way to learn what's to come so they can navigate their new normal together with their partner.

However, I also know that not all births and babies are the same. I've had friends who loved being pregnant, and those who experienced prenatal depression. I've had friends who went through their dream birth plans, and those who had to throw that plan in the trash as soon as they entered the hospital lobby. You never know what's going to happen in the delivery room, but that's just a small part of being a parent. I always compare the birth to the wedding. Many people hardly remember their weddings because they're so busy and in love, and let me tell you, giving birth is exactly the same! Weddings and births seem like huge deals in your mind, but they go by in a flash and then you're left navigating a new life with a new person. A wedding is fun, but the marriage is the part you're excited to devote yourself to. Similarly, giving birth is… well, I won't say it's fun, but it's certainly an experience. Then you've got an amazing child to devote yourself to.

That's where the comparisons end, because I'd argue that adapting to a marriage with another mature adult is much easier than starting from scratch with a newborn! But there's something equally exciting about becoming a parent that resembles what you feel as a newlywed. All the bliss and love tells you that your life has changed for the better. But there's definitely a learning curve with parenthood. And even if your partner has the pregnancy and birth experience of her dreams, postpartum is another beast altogether. She may have read all the books that tell her what will happen to her body and hormones, but what about you, the new dad? You're also going through a life change, wondering how to be the best parent while supporting your partner in whatever ways she needs.

Many new dads rely on their partner to tell them what she needs. When you're a couple, there's no problem with waiting for your partner to tell you what they need you to do to manage the workload and household chores. But when your partner is a new mother, she needs to focus on healing and caring for your newborn. It's your role to step up and care for your new family, pre-emptively giving your partner what she needs before she even realizes she needs it! How are you supposed to figure that out? Well, that's what this book will tell you!

I have years of experience as a lecturer, helping new parents adapt to life with their baby. I also coach couples one on one. I love sharing my research and experience with others, but also knew that those speaking engagements and personal appointments wouldn't help nearly as many people as a book would reach. So I opened a Word document and stared at the cursor for a bit before all my experiences and information came pouring out of me onto the page. I started by sharing a "best-case" scenario along with one that didn't go quite as planned. When it comes to pregnancy, labor, and postpartum, anything can happen. There aren't just two possible outcomes. But I wanted to highlight two in each chapter to help you see what I've helped couples navigate. Maybe an example will resemble your experience or maybe it won't, but you'll feel better knowing that there are many different options for each state of postpartum, instead of feeling like if you're not doing the best this researcher recommends, you're failing.

While I wrote this book with first-time fathers in mind, I must say that my husband and I used the advice each time we welcomed a new baby into our family. With each birth experience and baby being so different, it almost felt like starting from scratch. Referring back to what worked before gave us a jumping-off point, but we often had to change the advice slightly to suit our new family. I wanted to ensure that this book would help you and your partner regardless of your birth experience, family size, and baby's personality, so you'll want to keep this guidebook while your family expands.

I wish I could help all of you with one-on-one sessions to ensure I'm addressing your concerns, but since that's impossible, I've tried the next best thing! At the end of each chapter, there's a section of questions I'd ask you if we were together in a session. While I can't talk you through your answers, you'll get an idea of what to think about based on the information you've learned from the chapter. You'll be able to engage with the material and think about it in a way that applies to your personal situation.

Before we get started, I want to note that this book is intended to be inclusive of all partners entering parenthood. I love and accept all people, and want to support everyone on their journey of raising a child. However, for the simplicity of language, I will refer to the person who gave birth as the mother, partner, or wife, and the supporting partner will be the father, partner, or husband. But please know that this advice applies to everyone who is becoming a new parent, and I support you completely on this journey.

Let's get started!

Chapter 1:

What Is Postpartum?

One of my first clients was Sheri, a woman who had a doctor she loved and trusted, which made her look forward to her hospital birth. Sheri and her husband talked about what they wanted to do in case the medical professionals advised against her birth plan, so they had a backup that they felt comfortable with. They had all their bases covered for the worst-case scenario, but it turned out that labor went wonderfully. The mother and newborn were released from the hospital the day after the birth and the family was able to return home and settle into their new routine. I remember leaving their home after a visit to see how they'd adjusted, thinking, "This is why I got into the field!" Everything felt like it happened as it should.

About a year later, I worked with Marie and Todd, a couple who wanted a natural childbirth at home. They had a certified nurse midwife ready to help them inflate and fill a tub in their living room. Marie felt stressed by hospitals and knew she wanted to give birth in a place where she felt comfortable. Their backup plan was to use one of the water-birthing suites in the local hospital, since that room would give a similar vibe to their living room while still being in a hospital. However, the baby was breech, so a natural birth wasn't medically advisable. Marie got incredibly stressed at the idea of having a C-section in a traditional hospital room, which impacted her blood pressure and had negative impacts on both her and the baby. Though everything came out fine, it took Marie months to get past the trauma of not having her ideal birth. She felt guilty for her reaction to the unplanned surgery, while also harboring anger at herself and the medical professionals that a natural birth wasn't possible.

In both of these situations, the mothers had backup plans. They wanted one thing, but knew it might not happen. Above all, they wanted what was best for their babies. But you never know what may happen, even if you feel prepared and flexible. Even the most streamlined births can result in difficult postpartum periods. Understanding what will happen during this time will help you know how to support your partner.

Pregnancy and labor are clearly defined life experiences, with a beginning and end point. Postpartum is more loosely defined as "the transition back to prepregnancy state," but, as a mother, I have to say that's not really possible. Your body and life change so much after having a baby that you never truly go back to how you were before, physically, mentally, and emotionally.

The best way I can define postpartum, also called the postnatal period, is to call it the time following childbirth. That's as specific as you can get without cutting out certain groups or pushing women into the hole of perpetually being postpartum because they haven't returned to their "prepregnancy state." Your body goes through so many changes that you might never go back to your same size. Many women lose the weight gained during pregnancy but find their body has changed in other ways, so their old clothes still don't fit right! It can be frustrating, so I find that removing a specific definition from the term helps women cope with what they're experiencing.

That said, medical professionals define postpartum as six weeks. However, you should consider that medical professionals put a time limit on this period because of the need to schedule postpartum follow-up visits, so it's not on a strict timeline. Pregnancy lasts for three trimesters, ending when the woman gives birth. Therefore, most people consider the fourth trimester as a period of about three months, which is the definition I'll use for this book (Li et al., 1996).

Understanding what happens in the postpartum period will greatly help you know what your partner is going through and how you can support her.

A Comprehensive Look at the Fourth Trimester

The fourth trimester is just as involved as the trimesters of pregnancy. The mother will go through many physical, emotional, and hormonal changes that make it a difficult transition, because you're also adding a newborn into the mix. While the mother's body changes during pregnancy to accommodate the baby, the fourth trimester involves changing back to normal, such as the uterus contracting back to its typical size.

Understanding the Shift From Pregnancy to Postpartum

The shift from pregnancy to postpartum is a significant time for a woman. She's going from carrying a baby to caring for a newborn, plus handling all the physical and emotional changes that creates.

In terms of physical changes, her uterus is shrinking back to its previous size after growing with the baby. This causes lochia, which you'll read about in the next section.

Hormones necessary to help the baby grow inside your partner's body, like estrogen and progesterone, will decrease. However, her hormones don't level out because she'll have an increase of prolactin and oxytocin to promote breastfeeding. Breastfeeding is a subject on its own, which you'll read about in the next section.

Your partner may lose weight after giving birth to the baby and delivering the placenta, and some women lose weight while they're breastfeeding. However, not all do, so help your partner remember that not losing weight isn't a sign of failure, and there's no need to rush back to her prepregnancy size. Right now her focus should be eating enough to sustain herself and ensure she has the energy to physically heal and care for the baby.

Emotional changes vary based on your partner's history and home life. It's a major adjustment to become a parent, and many women experience baby blues in the first few weeks after childbirth. This period involves sadness, anxiety, irritability, and mood swings. Postpartum depression (PPD) also includes these symptoms, so we'll learn more about both in Chapter 3 to ensure you see the signs to best help your partner.

Needing to support a new human is emotionally taxing for both you and your partner. You will both probably experience sleep deprivation, too, which will impact you emotionally. I strongly recommend taking shifts with the baby, with one parent taking on the responsibility of care while the other rests, has a meal, hydrates, and can sit alone with their thoughts for a bit. I don't know about you, but my emotions run wild when I'm tired or hungry, even if there isn't a newborn in the picture, so prioritizing these simple aspects of self-care can really help you both stay emotionally balanced (Romano et al., 2010).

No matter what, bringing home a new baby is an adjustment that can make you and your partner have emotional reactions you wouldn't expect. Your family is growing, which is wonderful, but it changes your relationship with your partner, and it's okay to feel conflicted about that change. In fact, I think it's so serious that I've devoted Chapter 6 to the subject. So know that you'll learn more about how your relationship will change in time.

Common Postpartum Experiences

There are many common postpartum experiences women will face physically and emotionally.

Vaginal bleeding, or lochia, is a normal discharge of blood and uterine tissue after giving birth. It can last for a few weeks and shouldn't be confused with menstruation. Lochia rubra is the first stage, and is bright red and fairly heavy. It eases into lochia serosa, which is brown or pink. The final stage is lochia alba, which is pale yellow or white, more closely resembling vaginal discharge than blood. The progression of lochia helps your partner see that her body is healing after childbirth. The amount of lochia varies from woman to woman and can depend on the type of birth, such as vaginal or cesarean. Regardless of the circumstances, your partner should let the lochia flow from her body onto pads instead of using tampons, which can introduce bacteria into her uterus.

The mother's breasts also continue to change. Leading up to childbirth, they become engorged to prepare to feed the newborn. Once the baby is born, the milk comes in so the mother can breastfeed. Even if your partner doesn't plan to breastfeed, she'll have milk come in after giving birth. Her breasts may feel heavy, tender, or even painful. If she breastfeeds, she'll need to deal with the baby latching properly. Even effortless breastfeeding can cause cracked nipples and engorgement, and it demands a lot of the new mother's time, even if she pumps so you can bottle-feed the baby (Uludağ & Öztürk, 2020).

There are many other physical changes your partner will navigate, too. Due to hormonal changes, she may lose hair. This issue resolves itself in time, but it's still alarming to realize your hair is thinning on top of all the other changes happening at once. Body image is a major concern too. Even if a new mother feels healthy and loses weight, her body shape has most likely changed with pregnancy. This is a wonderful feature of the body—how it can change to grow and give birth to a new human! But when you're used to feeling one way, feeling another way can make it seem like you've completely lost yourself. And don't even get me started on what your partner sees when she looks in the mirror, and I'm not even solely talking about the spit-up on her shirt! Help her feel beautiful as she is—because she is!—during this time, because worrying about her appearance is an unnecessary stress in the fourth trimester. Comfort is key!

Hormones fluctuate all through your partner's pregnancy, which most likely led to a roller coaster of emotions for both of you. I'm sorry to say that won't end anytime soon. Her hormones changed to ensure her body could give the baby all it needed. Now that the baby is thriving independently, your partner's hormones need to balance back out to the levels she needs. Add into these fluctuations the idea that she's a new mother, caring for a baby, and feeling totally exhausted, and you might see her crying more than ever before, or perhaps getting angry at the drop of a hat. Give her space to feel these emotions and know things will level out in time.

While hormones greatly contribute to your partner's emotions, you should also keep an eye on her to see if she's going through the baby blues or something more severe, like PPD. We'll cover these in depth in Chapter 3 so you'll know exactly what to look for and how to get help for your partner.

Fatigue is something your partner will experience immediately after the Wonder Woman high of giving birth wears off. Don't feel left out—you'll experience it soon, if you aren't already. You'll have plenty of sleepless nights, but your partner is also experiencing fatigue from the stress of childbirth. Think about it: A baby came out of her body. She's a superhero! Let her rest, even if that means you're taking on all the housework or hiring someone to help out. Her physical recovery at this stage is crucial. After the stress of giving birth, there is so much potential for something to go wrong, so ensuring she can rest and relax is your most important role. Also check on her to ensure she's feeling okay, mentally and physically, and do whatever you must to guarantee she goes to all her follow-up appointments (Chauhan & Tadi, 2020).

The Partner's Role

The partner's role during the fourth trimester might often seem like you should take on as many chores as you can. While this is helpful for your partner, it can wear you out. You're much more beneficial if you're there to physically and emotionally support your wife in many ways, not just by completing chores. She'll need you to take on childcare, change diapers, and bond with the baby—as much for your sake as to give her a chance to shower and take a nap!

As your partner recovers, physically and emotionally, from giving birth, you'll need to provide emotional support and physical assistance in any way possible. You'll know exactly what you need to do based on your relationship with your partner. From your experience, if you know there are certain chores she hates, offer to take them on during this time. But you should try to be willing to take on cooking, cleaning, errands, and laundry to give your partner more time to heal. Or you can hire temporary help in terms of lawn care or cleaning. Order groceries instead of finding an hour to go to the store. Eat frozen meals or order takeout from your favorite restaurant. These changes don't have to be things you'll implement every month for the rest of your life, so consider splurging for a few months during the postpartum period to make everything easier on both of you (Dennis et al., 2017).

Emotional support is especially crucial. While it's true that both of you are new parents, only your wife went through childbirth. You may have let her squeeze your hand, but you don't know what her body went through to bring this child into the world. She may have loved giving birth, or she may grieve that she wasn't able to stick to her birth plan. Support her during this time, listening to her stories and encouraging her to share her feelings. It may feel tempting to brush away her worries since you have the baby in your arms right now, but feeling upset that things didn't go according to plan is incredibly valid, so listen to her with a nonjudgmental ear.

Emotional support doesn't only apply to your partner—you need to bond with the baby, too. You can help out your partner by taking the baby to spend time together, giving the new mom time to rest, shower, enjoy a meal uninterrupted, or catch up with her favorite show. Sometimes just giving her a chance to go for a solo drive or chat with a friend at a café can go a long way to helping her feel more like her usual self instead of "only" a mom, on demand whenever the baby needs her. Plus, spending time with your baby will help you feel more comfortable caring for them. You can feed them, change diapers, read stories, and sing nursery rhymes. Talk to your baby, watch their expressions, and rock them to sleep. Spending quality time together is a great foundation for a loving relationship with your child.

With all that said, it's not your job to do everything. While your partner's healing should be a priority for both of you, you also need to ensure you don't burn out. It's easy to try to take on everything to hold the family together, but that can be detrimental. Plus, there are some things you can't help with. If your wife feels depressed, don't placate her with inspirational quotes—encourage her to talk to her health-care provider, and do everything you can to ensure she attends follow-up appointments. If she's having trouble breastfeeding, help her find professional support like a lactation consultant or doula. You can also help with feeding by giving the baby bottles of pumped milk or formula to let your partner have a break.

Above all, just be there for your partner. Yes, you're both new parents, but you're still a couple that's very much in love. Make time for yourselves. Stay connected by talking about things other than the baby. Watch a movie together. Wait and cook dinner together after the baby goes to sleep. Hug, kiss, and hold hands. Make time to be alone together to ensure you keep your physical affection spark alive and satisfied.

Every family dynamic is different, so your role as partner may vary based on your relationship and what you and your spouse planned for parenting. As long as you're present, involved, and supportive during the fourth trimester, you'll be a great partner for the new mother. This is a transformative time, so being present will ensure you're helping to carry the load, though your role may change over time.

This list includes some of the ways I recommend new fathers support their partner during the fourth trimester:

- **Be present and attentive.** Be present and attentive to the new mother's needs. Offer emotional support and be ready to listen when she wants to talk about her feelings and experiences.

- **Help with household chores.** Take on household chores and responsibilities to relieve some of the burden from the new mother. Simple tasks like cooking, cleaning, and laundry can make a significant difference in reducing her stress.

- **Encourage rest and sleep.** The early days after childbirth can be exhausting for the new mother due to frequent feedings and caring for the baby. Encourage her to rest and take naps whenever possible, and offer to care for the baby during those times.

- **Assist with baby care.** Get involved in caring for the baby. Change diapers, bathe the baby, and offer to handle nighttime feedings to allow the new mother some much-needed rest. As a bonus, this extra engagement with your baby will help you bond with your child. You'll also learn how to take care of them in a trial by fire.

- **Educate yourself about postpartum recovery.** Learn about the physical and emotional changes that occur during the postpartum period. Understanding what the new mother is going through can help you provide more empathetic support. The first three chapters of this book help you understand what women may go through in childbirth, but also talk to your partner about the experience so you know exactly what she thought and felt during the process.

- **Provide healthy meals and snacks.** Nourishing the new mother with healthy meals and snacks is essential for her recovery and overall well-being. Prepare nutritious foods or arrange for meal deliveries.

- **Create a supportive environment.** Ensure that the home environment is supportive and conducive to the new mother's well-being. Dim the lights, play soothing music, and create a calm atmosphere to promote relaxation.

- **Celebrate her accomplishments.** Acknowledge and celebrate the new mother's accomplishments, no matter how small they may seem. Compliments and words of encouragement can boost her confidence as a new parent.

- **Offer gentle affection.** Offer physical affection, such as hugs and cuddles, to show your love and support. Physical touch can be comforting and reassuring during this time.

- **Encourage self-care.** Remind the new mother to take care of herself. Encourage her to engage in self-care activities like taking a warm bath, reading a book, or spending some time alone.

- **Communicate openly.** Encourage open communication between you and the new mother. Be willing to listen and express your feelings as well.

- **Handle visitors and requests.** Shield the new mother from overwhelming visitors or external demands during the early postpartum period. Help manage visitors' expectations and prioritize her needs.

- **Be patient and understanding.** Postpartum recovery can be a roller coaster of emotions. Be patient and understanding, and avoid putting pressure on the new mother to "bounce back" too quickly.

- **Assist with breastfeeding.** If the new mother is breastfeeding, offer support by learning about breastfeeding techniques, helping with positioning, and providing water and snacks during feeding sessions.

- **Take care of yourself.** Don't forget to take care of yourself too. Supporting a new mother can be emotionally and physically demanding, so make sure you get enough rest and find ways to recharge.

By providing thoughtful and compassionate support, dads play a vital role in helping new mothers recover from childbirth and adjust to the demands of parenthood. Your love, understanding, and assistance during this time can foster a strong bond between you as parents and create a positive foundation for your growing family.

In Our Session

If we were having a one-on-one session about the postpartum experience, there are a few questions I'd ask you to see how you were feeling about this aspect of your life:

- How do you view your role as a father in relation to your partner's role as a mother? How has this perception evolved since the baby's arrival?

- What were your expectations about fatherhood before the baby was born, and how have those expectations shifted?

- How are you managing the balance between your role as a partner and your role as a father?

- Are there any specific challenges you've encountered while adjusting to your new role? How have you been addressing these challenges?

Chapter 2:

Physical Health

My client Sarah came out of her natural labor feeling like it was nothing, thanks to the high of holding her brand-new baby in her arms after giving birth. However, that emotional joy she felt when she was around her baby devolved into physical pain and soreness when she didn't have the distraction of her daughter. She had a few stitches due to some minor tears and knew she needed to clean them carefully with her perineal squirt bottle. Her doctor also recommended she soak pads in witch hazel and pop them in the freezer for a cool compression against her stitches. However, Sarah was used to being active, so sitting around made her feel like she couldn't do anything on her own. Her partner took on extra household chores and encouraged Sarah to bond with her baby while also drinking plenty of water, eating a healthy diet, and resting. After a few weeks, Sarah was able to take short walks around the neighborhood, and eventually got back to doing gentle exercises as her stitches healed.

Jessica was a client who had a cesarean birth. She knew there were risks with her pregnancy before she and her husband conceived, so she accepted the birth plan. What she didn't realize, however, was how much pain she'd feel at the incision site. Jessica told me she felt like she had been chopped in half and clumsily put back together! She could hold and nurse her baby fine, but picking up the baby hurt, and she couldn't cook or clean without the pain overwhelming her. Though she hated asking for help, Jessica asked her partner to take on more chores. Both her mother and mother-in-law took turns coming over to cook, clean, and visit the baby while Jessica rested. When her doctor said she was ready, Jessica started light exercises, even though she was so scared of reopening the wound. However, her baby inspired her to continue healing and rebuilding her strength so she could get back to her full health and be the best mother for her baby.

These stories are important to consider because many people think of the impact of postpartum hormones on emotional health during this time, but disregard physical health. Whether your partner has a vaginal or cesarean birth, her body has a lot of healing to do. While you might think of tearing, soreness, and C-section wounds, there are other physical issues that also require rest and recovery.

Common Occurrences in Labor

Throughout pregnancy, a woman's body changes to accommodate the developing baby, while also making changes to ensure her body is ready for birth. The cervix thins out, the hips expand, and the joints loosen. However, even if your partner's body prepares for labor, things might not go smoothly. Every body is different, but there are some common occurrences in both vaginal and cesarean births for you to be aware of.

Vaginal Birth

A vaginal birth, also known as a natural or normal birth, is the process of delivering a baby through the birth canal, or vagina, without the need for surgical intervention. During a vaginal birth, the baby passes through the cervix and vagina to be born into the world. It's the most common method of childbirth for women with low-risk pregnancies and when there are no medical indications for a cesarean (C-section).

There are five distinct stages of labor:

1. **Early labor.** This is the initial phase of labor when contractions begin and the cervix starts to dilate and efface.

2. **Active labor.** As labor progresses, the contractions become more intense and regular. The cervix continues to dilate, allowing the baby to descend further into the birth canal.

3. **Transition.** This is the most intense phase of labor as the cervix is fully dilated, typically at 10 centimeters. Women may

experience strong contractions and intense pressure during this stage.

4. **Pushing and birth.** Once the cervix is fully dilated, the woman is encouraged to push with each contraction to help the baby move through the birth canal. With each push, the baby's head advances until it crowns, or becomes visible at the vaginal opening. The baby's head is then delivered, followed by the rest of their body.

5. **Placenta delivery.** After the baby is born, the placenta, which provides nourishment to the baby during pregnancy, needs to be delivered. This usually happens shortly after the baby is born.

In the early stages of a vaginal birth, your partner will experience contractions to dilate the cervix. The uterine muscles contract to move the baby through the birth canal. As the body prepares for birth and the baby gets ready, the contractions become more intense in terms of both pain and duration. They will also start occurring more closely together, so some women can hardly catch their breath before another contraction makes them double over in pain. Other discomforts like back pain, cramps, and pelvic pressure can happen during contractions.

Some women experience their water breaking. This is actually the amniotic sac rupturing, releasing amniotic fluid, which resembles water. However, some women are ready to give birth without their water breaking, and the amniotic sac will rupture during labor. If not, the medical professional can rupture the sac for them. Throughout labor, the baby's heart rate and the mother's contractions are usually monitored to ensure the baby's well-being.

During contractions, which are part of active labor, women can manage pain with breathing exercises. They can also change positions, with some women preferring to stand or walk through the pain, while others may sit on a birthing ball or get on their hands and knees to reduce back pressure. The cervix, the lower part of the uterus, needs to dilate, or open, and efface, or thin out, to allow the baby to pass through the birth canal. Cervical dilation is measured in centimeters, and effacement is measured in percentages.

By the time the cervix is 10 centimeters dilated, the mother will be ready to push the baby through the birth canal and into the world. When the cervix is fully dilated and the baby's head is low enough in the birth canal, the woman is encouraged to push during contractions to assist the baby's passage through the vagina. As the baby's head descends through the birth canal, it may become visible at the vaginal opening during contractions. This is known as crowning and is an exciting moment as the baby's arrival is near. Depending on your preferred level of involvement and type of birth, some medical professionals allow the parents to gently touch the baby's head during crowning. Once the baby is born, the placenta needs to be delivered. After the delivery of the placenta, the woman may experience uterine contractions, often called afterbirth pains, as the uterus returns to its prepregnancy size.

Regardless of how the birth progresses, there are a few common side effects from vaginal birth. Many women experience perineal soreness and swelling. The perineum is the area between the vagina and anus, which can stretch or tear as the baby makes its way out of your partner's body. This type of stress on that area can make it swell, bruise, or stay sore for several weeks, which can make it difficult for your partner to sit or walk.

An episiotomy is a surgical cut made to widen the vaginal opening to help the baby out. Like vaginal tears, there are stitches involved with an episiotomy to ensure healing. Your partner will need to gently clean the area to keep it from becoming infected as it heals (Desai & Tsukerman, 2021).

Vaginal births have various potential advantages, including quicker recovery times, decreased infection risks, and improved bonding between the mother and the infant. However, not all pregnancies are suited for vaginal birth, and some women may require a cesarean section for a variety of medical reasons, including fetal distress, placenta previa, or certain maternal health issues.

Pregnant women should discuss their birth preferences, as well as any potential medical concerns, with their health-care providers in order to select the safest and most appropriate birthing method for their specific circumstances. The ultimate purpose of childbirth is to ensure the mother's and baby's well-being and health.

Cesarean Birth

Women can plan a cesarean birth, or it can happen if they have dystocia, which is a difficult birth like a breech baby or where there is fetal distress or health concerns about the baby or mother (Shields et al., 2007). Whether planned or simply necessary, a cesarean is a surgical procedure that involves making an incision in the abdominal wall and uterus to retrieve the baby.

Because it's a surgical procedure, mothers receive regional anesthesia, like an epidural or spinal block, to numb the lower half of their body. However, the mother remains awake and alert during the process. The medical professionals will either make a horizontal incision, called a "bikini cut," or a vertical incision, called the "classic cut," in the mother's lower abdomen to access the uterus.

Once the uterus is opened, the baby is gently delivered through the incision. The baby is then carefully handed over to the medical team for evaluation and care. The mother may feel tugging or pressure as the medical team reaches the baby. After the baby is out, the medical professionals will stitch up the wound with sutures or staples and give the mother time to bond with her newborn.

Throughout the procedure, the mother's vital signs, such as heart rate, blood pressure, and oxygen levels, are closely monitored. The anesthesia is also managed to ensure the mother's comfort and safety during the surgery. Following the surgery, the mother is taken to a recovery area where she can be closely monitored as the anesthesia wears off. Pain management and wound care are provided during this time. Breastfeeding can still be initiated after a C-section, but it might be delayed due to the mother's recovery and the use of anesthesia, so the medical providers can give more advice about this situation.

While mother and baby can leave anywhere from 24 to 48 hours after a vaginal birth, a woman who experiences a cesarean may have to stay in the hospital for several days. The medical team will check in to ensure she's starting the healing process. The additional time in the hospital will also help her understand how easy she needs to take things once she's home to prevent reopening the wound. A scar will form at the incision site, which may take time to heal and fade. Following proper wound care instructions is essential to minimize scarring and promote healing.

Vaginal births lead to a certain type of discomfort and pain, but cesarean births are a whole different can of worms. Women still have soreness from pregnancy, but they're also handling surgical wounds. A C-section cuts through skin, muscle, and the uterus, so there's a lot to heal. It can hurt to laugh and cough, and moving can take time and effort. It's hard to stretch, reach, or lift things due to the position of the incision, so mothers need to take it easy and follow all recommended postoperative advice from their medical team (Martin et al., 2017). Mothers who undergo a cesarean birth may experience a range of emotions, including relief that the baby is safe, but also disappointment or sadness about not having a vaginal birth.

It's important to remember that a cesarean birth is a major surgery and carries its own set of risks and benefits. Medical professionals carefully assess the need for a C-section and discuss the procedure with the expectant mother before making any decisions. The goal is always to ensure the safety and well-being of both the mother and the baby.

Potential Birth Complications

Birth is a miraculous and natural process, but it can also be accompanied by various potential complications that may pose challenges for both the mother and the baby. While many births proceed smoothly, there are instances where unforeseen medical issues arise, requiring swift and specialized interventions. These complications can arise due to factors such as premature birth, maternal health conditions, fetal distress, or unforeseen birth abnormalities. In this context, it becomes crucial for health-care professionals to be vigilant and prepared to address any complications that may arise during childbirth, ensuring the best possible outcome for both mother and baby. Understanding the potential birth complications can aid in early recognition, timely interventions, and compassionate care, promoting the health and well-being of all involved parties. Knowing the possibilities will also help you be more prepared for what you may encounter once your baby is born. All parents want a smooth birth with a healthy baby, but that's not always the case. Having information puts you in a better position to adjust to any changes without the additional stress of learning everything while you're already immersed in it.

Neonatal Intensive Care Unit Stays

If a baby is born prematurely or with certain medical conditions, they may need to be admitted to the neonatal intensive care unit (NICU) for specialized monitoring and treatment. The NICU provides round-the-clock care from a team of health-care professionals experienced in handling newborns with complex medical needs. There are many reasons why your medical team may want to keep your baby in the NICU.

Babies born weighing less than 5.5 pounds may be considered low birth weight. These infants might need extra care and monitoring to ensure they are growing and developing properly. Premature babies, or babies born before 37 weeks of gestation, often need NICU care because their organs, especially the lungs, may not be fully developed. This makes it difficult for them to breathe and regulate their body temperature on their own.

In some cases, babies may experience birth injuries, such as fractures, nerve injuries, or bruising, which might necessitate specialized care. Babies born with infections or those who develop infections shortly after birth may need treatment in the NICU. Other birth complications, such as meconium aspiration syndrome, which happens when a baby inhales their first stool, or birth asphyxia, which is the failure to breathe independently at birth, may necessitate NICU care (Sayad & Silva-Carmona, 2020).

Some babies may have difficulty breathing after birth due to underdeveloped lungs, infection, or other factors. They may require respiratory support, such as oxygen therapy or mechanical ventilation (Neonatal Intensive Care Unit [NICU]: Common Problems, 2017).

The NICU is equipped with specialized medical equipment, skilled health-care professionals, and an environment tailored to meet the unique needs of newborns with medical complexities. The length of stay in the NICU varies depending on the baby's condition and how they respond to treatment. Health-care providers strive to offer the best care possible to help these babies grow and develop so they can eventually be discharged and go home with their families.

The exact process will vary depending on your baby's health, but in general, NICU visits start with a medical assessment. The medical team will thoroughly check vital signs, perform diagnostic tests, and assess any specific medical concerns. Based on the assessment, a personalized care plan will be developed for your baby. This plan will outline the medical treatments, interventions, and procedures required for their specific needs. The NICU is equipped with advanced medical technology and specialized equipment to care for premature and critically ill newborns. This may include incubators, ventilators, monitors, feeding tubes, and other medical devices.

Babies in the NICU are continuously monitored to track vital signs, oxygen levels, heart rate, breathing, and other essential parameters. This continuous monitoring helps detect any changes or concerns promptly. Depending on your baby's condition, they may receive specialized feeding techniques through either a feeding tube or breastfeeding, if possible. Nutrition is closely monitored to support your baby's growth and development. If necessary, your baby will receive medications and treatments to address specific medical issues, administered by the medical team according to the prescribed schedule.

The NICU staff works closely with various specialists, such as neonatologists, pediatricians, nurses, respiratory therapists, and other health-care professionals, to ensure comprehensive care for your baby.

While you can feel confident that your baby is in good hands while they stay in the NICU for treatment, you might not feel as comfortable. It's an emotional time, so you'll likely feel stressed and not know how to cope.

First of all, establish open and honest communication with the NICU staff. Ask questions about your baby's condition, treatment plan, and progress. Understanding what is happening can alleviate anxiety. Learning about the equipment, procedures, and medical terminology can make the NICU environment feel less overwhelming (Ringley, 2021). Request regular updates from the NICU staff if you are unable to be with your baby all the time. Knowing your baby's progress can provide some reassurance. However, maintain a careful balance. You don't want to research too much and start expecting the worst. Just as you can choose any lone symptom, look it up on WebMD, and get a death sentence, you can find out too much information that won't be helpful for you. It's better to have a basic knowledge of the situation and then ask for realistic information from the medical professionals instead of attempting to get to the root of the problem yourself.

While you balance your research and medical questions with reality, you should also reach out to family, friends, or support groups to share your feelings and concerns. Talking to others who have gone through a similar experience can be comforting and help you feel less isolated. In my experience with clients, talking about NICU stays is almost as rare as talking about PPD and other mood disorders. There's no shame in your baby staying in the NICU, but many mothers think that their body failed them by not providing their baby with everything necessary. Instead of letting these thoughts overwhelm you, know that medical professionals are trained for these situations and do everything they can to help your baby heal to their best selves. If you're open about your experience, you might be surprised to find how many other parents have gone through something similar.

When your baby is in the NICU, it may seem like your real life stops. But you can take action to try and make it seem more normal. Participate in tasks such as diaper changes, feeding (if possible), and skin-to-skin contact when allowed. This can strengthen your bond with your baby and provide comfort (Coping with the Neonatal Intensive Care Unit [NICU]: Tips, n.d.). You'll also be able to start adjusting to parenthood as you'll need to when you bring your baby home. While you'll be in the hospital instead of your cozy home, you can still start getting the feel for feeding, changing, and holding your baby. Ask your medical team to be sure, but some hospitals allow parents to bring in baby blankets and baby clothes so they can be reminded of how they prepared for their baby. You can also bring stuffed animals, though they'll just be near your baby, not in bed with them, for safety reasons. You can also bring family pictures to tape to the incubator for your baby to have loved ones nearby at all times. Your NICU stay will be a temporary stop, but there's no reason you shouldn't ask for the ability to make this area a little more cozy for your baby, you, and your wife.

Although it's difficult, try to maintain a positive outlook. The NICU staff are trained to provide the best care possible, and many babies do make a full recovery and go home. Strive to celebrate each small step of progress your baby makes. It can help focus on positive moments amid the challenging experience. It may feel difficult to think positively when your whole life is up in the air, but you'll appreciate the opportunity to look back on these experiences once you're past them. It's a major growing experience for you, your partner, and your baby. With that said, you shouldn't brush off your negative emotions. You're not wrong to feel sad or scared that your baby is in the NICU. Medical stress is so uncertain that no one will judge you for being upset, so don't judge yourself for it, either. As long as you don't wallow in these feelings and let them take over, you can acknowledge them before letting them go in favor of positivity.

It's okay to take breaks from the NICU if you need to rest or recharge. Ensure that there is someone you trust to stay with your baby during these times. You might find that writing about your experiences, feelings, and emotions can be cathartic and help you process your emotions.

Know that managing life outside of the NICU can be challenging. Don't hesitate to ask for help with household chores, errands, and other responsibilities. If you find it challenging to cope, consider speaking with a counselor, therapist, or social worker who has experience in NICU-related issues (Novak, 2022).

Every NICU journey is unique, and it's essential to be patient with yourself and your emotions. Celebrate the progress your baby makes, no matter how small, and have faith in the expertise of the medical team caring for your little one. Remember that your partner is going through the same thing, so you can both support and encourage each other. You want to rely on each other and come together at this time, so don't let the stress or frustrations push you apart.

When your baby's condition improves, and they are stable, the medical team will work with you to prepare for your baby's transition home. They will provide guidance on care routines, feeding, and any necessary medical follow-up. The process may look different from what you imagined when you grabbed your wife's hospital bag just days or weeks ago, but you'll get to bring your baby home and transition to your new life as a family of three.

Jaundice

Jaundice is a medical disorder that causes the skin, the mucous membranes, and the whites of the eyes to turn yellow. It happens when there's too much bilirubin in the bloodstream. Bilirubin is a yellow pigment that's created naturally during the breakdown of red blood cells. Neonatal jaundice is what some babies may experience in their first few days of life. It's usually a temporary situation that won't cause long-term harm, but in some cases it may lead to complications.

In severe cases of untreated or inadequately managed jaundice, high levels of bilirubin can cross the blood–brain barrier and lead to a condition called kernicterus. Kernicterus is a rare but serious neurological disorder that can cause permanent brain damage, hearing loss, and developmental delays. Bilirubin encephalopathy is another term for kernicterus, referring to the neurological complications caused by high levels of bilirubin in the brain. High bilirubin levels can affect the ability of the baby's liver to produce glucose, leading to low blood sugar levels, known as hypoglycemia (Mishra et al., 2008).

Jaundiced babies may become lethargic and have difficulty feeding, which can lead to dehydration and weight loss. Severe jaundice can weaken the baby's immune system, making them more susceptible to infections. If jaundice leads to kernicterus or severe brain damage, it can result in long-term developmental issues, including cognitive and motor impairments (Newman et al., 1990).

Closely monitor your newborn for jaundice, especially in their first week of life. In many cases, mild jaundice resolves on its own without any intervention. However, if the jaundice is more severe or persists, medical professionals may recommend treatments such as phototherapy, which is exposure to special lights that help break down bilirubin.

In rare cases, they may arrange an exchange transfusion, where they replace the baby's blood with donor blood to lower bilirubin levels and prevent complications. The baby is placed under special blue or white lights that help break down the excess bilirubin in the skin. The baby may wear only a diaper and protective eye patches during phototherapy sessions. Phototherapy is usually well-tolerated and has minimal side effects.

Encouraging the baby to feed more frequently can help increase bowel movements, which aids in the elimination of bilirubin from the body. In cases where the baby is not feeding well and there is a risk of dehydration or low blood sugar, supplemental feeding with expressed breast milk or formula may be recommended.

If the jaundice is due to an underlying medical condition, such as an infection or a blood disorder, the medical professionals will treat your baby for the primary cause.

You should always consult with your health-care provider if you notice any signs of jaundice in your newborn, such as yellowing of the skin or eyes, to ensure appropriate evaluation and management. Early detection and proper treatment can significantly reduce the risk of complications associated with neonatal jaundice.

Vision and Hearing Issues

Babies can experience various hearing and vision issues, some of which may be present at birth (congenital) or develop shortly after. Early detection and intervention are crucial for addressing these issues effectively. Hearing and vision screening for newborns is usually done in the hospital or birthing center shortly after birth. Early detection allows for early intervention in cases where difficulties are discovered, which can dramatically improve outcomes for babies with hearing and vision problems. You should make sure that your newborn undergoes these screening tests as part of their normal postnatal care. If you have concerns about your baby's hearing or eyesight, you should discuss these with your health-care professional for additional evaluation. There are noninvasive tests and screenings for your newborn that will alert you to these issues.

The otoacoustic emissions (OAE) test assesses the inner ear's (cochlea) sensitivity to sound. A tiny probe with a microphone is inserted into the baby's ear, and noises are played back. If the cochlea of the newborn is functioning properly, an echo response (otoacoustic emission) is produced and recorded by the microphone (Your Baby's Hearing Screening and Next Steps, 2021). The auditory brainstem response (ABR) test records electrical activity generated by the auditory nerve and brainstem to assess the brain's response to sound. While clicking noises are provided through headphones or speakers, electrodes are implanted on the baby's skull (Newborn Hearing Screening, 2020).

To check your newborn's vision, the optician will shine a light into the baby's eyes to perform a red reflex test. When light reflects off the retina, the red reflex should appear as a red glow in the center of the eye. This aids in the detection of potential eye problems such as cataracts or retinoblastoma. The optician may also conduct a pupil response test, which examines the response of the baby's pupils to light. To observe the baby's pupils, a penlight or flashlight is utilized, and the pupils should contract in reaction to the light (Jullien, 2021).

Remember that these are screening tests, not diagnostic examinations. If any problems are discovered during the screening, more examinations and testing may be required to confirm the findings and identify the best course of action.

Some hearing issues you may experience include:

- **Congenital hearing loss.** Due to hereditary reasons, infections during pregnancy, or other unknown causes, some babies are born deaf.

- **Otitis media.** This is a common ear infection that can temporarily impair your baby's hearing. It happens when the middle ear becomes inflamed and filled with fluid.

- **Auditory neuropathy spectrum disorder (ANSD).** ANSD is a condition in which sound is processed incorrectly in the auditory nerve, resulting in hearing problems.

- **Hearing loss due to prematurity.** Premature babies may be more susceptible to hearing loss due to a variety of causes, including drug exposure or mechanical ventilation.

- **Noise-induced hearing loss.** Prolonged exposure to loud noises can damage a baby's hearing (Wroblewska-Seniuk et al., 2016).

Some vision issues your baby may have include:

- **Refractive errors.** Blurred vision in newborns can be caused by refractive abnormalities such as nearsightedness, farsightedness, and astigmatism.

- **Strabismus (crossed eyes).** Strabismus is a condition in which the eyes are not correctly aligned, resulting in crossed or misaligned eyes.

- **Amblyopia (lazy eye).** Due to a lack of visual stimulation, one eye develops greater vision than the other, resulting in amblyopia. Amblyopia, if not treated promptly, can result in irreversible visual loss in the affected eye.

- **Congenital cataracts.** Cataracts are clouding of the lens of the eye and can occur at birth or develop later in life. Congenital cataracts can cause vision impairment or blindness if left untreated.

- **Retinopathy of prematurity (ROP).** ROP, or abnormal blood vessel growth in the retina, is a risk for premature babies. Severe occurrences can result in blindness or vision loss.

- **Coloboma.** Coloboma is a disorder that causes a gap or hole in one or more eye structures, such as the iris, retina, or optic nerve (de Aguiar et al., 2011).

You can check on your baby's hearing and vision in addition to taking these screening measures. If your baby has a hearing issue, you may notice that they don't startle when they're near a loud noise. They may not respond to your voice, while most babies will turn toward their parents' voices by the time they're a few months old. They may also have delayed speech and language development. Your baby should start cooing as soon as they discover their voice, and will have "conversations" with you when you talk back. If this doesn't happen, the delay may mean they can't hear well. You can also see if your baby is inattentive or unresponsive to sounds around them. Instead of being focused on what they're doing, they may be unable to hear.

Vision issues are something else you can watch for. You might see abnormal eye movements, like if your baby's eyes wander a lot or get crossed. They may also keep their eyes closed often or squint, which demonstrates a sensitivity to light that can be related to vision problems. White or gray pupils instead of black could be a visual sign of cataracts. By the time they're a couple of months old, your baby should be making eye contact with you. If they don't, or seem disinterested in faces, whether real or in photographs and books, it may be a vision problem. Around this time they will also visually track objects and people. You can hold up an object and move it slowly back and forth to see if their eyes follow it. If not, they may have visual impairments.

These are just a few ideas of what to look for in terms of hearing and vision issues. But not all babies will show the same signals, and some of these behaviors may be normal for particular developmental periods. However, if you detect any chronic or concerning hearing or vision symptoms, get further opinions from a pediatrician, audiologist, or eye-care specialist. Early detection and intervention are important for addressing potential problems and encouraging healthy infant development. Regular medical checkups can help monitor your baby's overall health and development, including their hearing and eyesight.

Treatment for hearing and vision issues will help your baby experience all the sights and sounds of the world. If your baby has hearing issues, your medical team may suggest that they wear hearing aids to help them hear sounds. In cases of profound hearing loss, specialists may recommend cochlear implants. These are surgically implanted devices that stimulate the auditory nerve directly. They will help the baby perceive sound at most volumes. Auditory–verbal therapy can assist children with hearing loss by improving their skills relating to listening and spoken language (Wroblewska-Seniuk et al., 2016). Depending on the results of the hearing tests, your medical team can recommend that your family works with a speech–language pathologist or audiologist to benefit your child's hearing, language, and communication. Early intervention programs that support and guide families in developing their child's speech and language development may benefit babies with hearing loss.

For refractive vision issues, your baby may wear prescription glasses. Some eye conditions, like strabismus and congenital cataracts, may require surgery to improve your baby's vision. Vision therapy is another option, involving a set of exercises and activities designed to improve various visual skills and talents. Eye patches may be used to cover the stronger eye in babies with amblyopia (lazy eye), causing the weaker eye to work harder and develop improved vision. To treat underlying issues such as infections or inflammation, eye drops or ointments may be administered.

Health-care professionals will establish a specific treatment plan based on the baby's diagnosis, age, overall health, and the severity of the ailment. To ensure the best possible care and support for their infant, parents must collaborate closely with their child's health-care providers, audiologists, and eye-care specialists.

Regular check-ins and ongoing monitoring are essential for assessing progress and making any required changes to the treatment plan. Many babies with hearing and vision problems can have excellent outcomes and attain their developmental potential with adequate intervention and support.

Feeding Issues

Babies might have a variety of eating concerns, which can be difficult for both the baby and the parents. Feeding problems can occur for a variety of reasons, including medical ailments, developmental issues, or behavioral issues.

Breastfeeding can be difficult for some babies due to latching issues, a poor sucking response, or insufficient milk production from the mother. Some babies may have bottle-feeding issues, such as nipple confusion, swallowing, or excessive spitting up. Some babies may exhibit aversion or unwillingness to eat due to sensory difficulties, discomfort, or medical disorders. Babies who do not get enough nutrition or who have feeding problems may struggle with weight gain, which is worrying for their general health and development (Bernard-Bonnin, 2006).

Gastroesophageal reflux disease (GERD) is a condition in which stomach contents flow back into the esophagus, producing discomfort and agitation while eating meals or breastfeeding. Some babies may acquire food allergies or intolerances, resulting in digestive disorders and feeding difficulties.

Breastfeeding or bottle-feeding becomes difficult when the baby's tongue or lip is too closely linked to the mouth's floor or upper lip. A tongue tie restricts the range of motion of a baby's tongue, while a lip tie is a condition that restricts the space between a baby's upper and lower gums. Similarly, babies who have oral motor issues may struggle to coordinate the motions required for sucking, swallowing, and feeding.

Due to underdeveloped sucking and swallowing reflexes, premature newborns may have difficulty feeding. Feeding problems are sometimes associated with behavioral concerns, such as distractibility or an unwillingness to eat owing to preferences.

Parents should keep an eye on their baby's feeding habits and behavior, especially during the first year of life. If you observe any recurrent feeding problems or have concerns about your baby's nutrition and growth, see a pediatrician or a feeding specialist. Early detection and intervention can assist in addressing feeding issues and ensuring that your baby receives the necessary assistance for healthy growth and development. Feeding problems are typically manageable with the correct assistance, and health-care professionals can provide tailored advice and solutions to meet your baby's individual requirements (Rodriguez, 2019).

Treatment for feeding problems in babies is determined by the underlying reason as well as the specific feeding difficulties the baby is experiencing. To design a specific treatment plan, collaborate closely with a health-care expert, such as a pediatrician or a feeding specialist. For breastfeeding difficulties, a lactation consultant can provide guidance on proper positioning and latching techniques to ensure effective breastfeeding. Feeding therapists, speech–language pathologists, or occupational therapists can work with the baby to address oral motor difficulties and improve feeding skills. For babies with GERD, the doctor may recommend lifestyle changes, positioning techniques, or medications to manage the reflux. If a tongue or lip tie causes feeding difficulties, a medical procedure known as a frenectomy may be performed. This will release the tight tissue and improve the baby's ability to feed.

You can try a few things on your own, like using different bottle types or nipple shapes to help babies who experience bottle-feeding difficulties. If the baby has food allergies or intolerances, eliminating the triggering foods from the mother's diet in the case of breastfeeding or using specialized hypoallergenic formulas may be necessary. Establishing a feeding schedule and ensuring proper pacing during feeds can be helpful for babies who are overwhelmed or resistant during feedings. In cases where the baby isn't gaining enough weight, the doctor may recommend supplemental feeding with expressed breast milk or formula to ensure adequate nutrition (Fischer, 2022).

You should talk honestly with your health-care providers about your baby's feeding problems, since this will help with the development of an effective treatment plan. Feeding problems can be stressful for both the baby and the parents, so seeking help and advice from health-care practitioners, feeding specialists, and support groups can be helpful.

You might feel helpless when your baby isn't eating right or getting enough nutrition, but keeping a level head and seeking professional support can make all the difference.

Post-Labor Experiences

Post-labor experiences encompass a wide range of physical, emotional, and psychological changes that women undergo in the aftermath of childbirth. As the body begins to heal and adjust to its postpartum state, women may encounter various unique challenges and joys that define their initial days, weeks, and months as new mothers. From the tender moments of bonding with their newborn to the physical recovery and hormonal fluctuations, post-labor experiences shape the foundation of motherhood, offering a profound and life-changing chapter in a woman's life. This section covers some common post-labor experiences, shedding light on the diverse and extraordinary path to embracing motherhood.

Physical Recovery

The postpartum period involves physical healing from childbirth. This includes the uterus shrinking back to its prepregnancy size, healing of any perineal tears or incisions in the case of either a vaginal birth or a C-section, and the body gradually returning to its prepregnancy state. The length of physical recovery after childbirth can vary for each woman and depends on several factors, including the type of birth, the overall health of the mother, and any complications experienced during childbirth.

For women who had a vaginal birth without significant complications or tearing, the initial physical recovery typically takes about four to six weeks. During this time, the uterus contracts back to its prepregnancy size, vaginal bleeding decreases and stops, and any perineal discomfort or swelling resolves. However, some women may still experience lingering discomfort or soreness beyond the initial recovery period.

Recovery after a cesarean birth usually takes longer compared to vaginal birth. The initial recovery period is about six to eight weeks. During this time, the incision site heals and the mother gradually regains strength and mobility. It's important to follow the health-care provider's guidelines for wound care and activity restrictions to promote proper healing.

Bleeding and Clotting

Women have bleeding after giving birth, regardless of which method of labor they experienced. As mentioned in Chapter 1, lochia happens after both vaginal and cesarean births, as the uterus sloughs off its lining and releases blood, mucus, and tissue (Stranges et al., 2012). Postpartum bleeding starts after childbirth and can last several weeks, until the uterus completely sheds the lining.

Clotting can naturally happen in lochia, so you shouldn't feel alarmed unless the clots aren't a reasonable size. Lochia will coagulate and form small clots, from specks to the size of a grape. If they are bigger than a golf ball or accompany excessive bleeding, you should contact your partner's medical team for advice (Watson, 2020).

Perineal Discomfort

Women who have had vaginal births may experience perineal discomfort or soreness, especially if they had a tear or episiotomy. Warm sitz baths, pain-relief medications, and proper wound care can help alleviate discomfort.

Constipation

Many women experience constipation after giving birth due to hormonal changes and dehydration. The body needs plenty of fluid to dispose of waste, so drinking water will help solve this problem. However, some women are on pain medication after giving birth, especially if it was a C-section or involved an episiotomy. Some medications have constipation as a side effect.

Whether or not your partner experiences constipation for these reasons, she may feel too worried to push during a bowel movement. It can feel precarious if she has stitches in the perineal area. Hemorrhoids are also common experiences post-labor. The strain from pushing during childbirth can cause hemorrhoids or make them worse, which can make it painful to have a bowel movement (Watson, 2020).

Incontinence

Women who push during labor may have pelvic floor issues that can cause temporary urinary incontinence. They don't have complete control over their bladder during this time, so they may leak when they sneeze, cough, or laugh. A medical professional will recommend exercises, like Kegels, to strengthen your partner's pelvic floor and help them overcome incontinence (Letko, 2019).

Breast Changes

After childbirth, the breasts start producing milk. Women may experience breast engorgement, tenderness, or leakage as their bodies adjust to breastfeeding or if they choose to formula-feed.

For women who choose to breastfeed, their breasts may experience engorgement and tenderness during the first few weeks. As the breasts adjust to breastfeeding, they may feel tender, especially during the first few weeks. This tenderness usually improves as breastfeeding becomes more established. When a baby starts feeding or even when a mother thinks about her baby, the letdown reflex can be triggered. This is a response that causes milk to flow from the breast ducts and be available for the baby to consume. Establishing a breastfeeding routine can take time, and some women may experience sore nipples or discomfort during this period, but making time to breastfeed or pump can alleviate much of the discomfort.

If a woman does not breastfeed after childbirth, her breasts will still undergo certain changes during the postpartum period. However, these changes will be different compared to the changes experienced by a woman who breastfeeds. In the first few days after childbirth, the breasts may become engorged as they prepare for milk production. However, without breastfeeding, the milk production will gradually decrease, and the engorgement should resolve within a week or so. For women who do not breastfeed, the milk production will be naturally suppressed over time. The hormone prolactin, responsible for milk production, will gradually decrease as there is no demand for breastfeeding. After childbirth, breast size may decrease as the milk production ceases and the breasts return to their prepregnancy size. This process can take a few weeks to a few months, depending on the woman.

Hormonal Changes

Hormones change during pregnancy to support the growing baby while also ensuring your partner's body is ready to give birth. This means that they need to recalibrate after giving birth. After the baby is born, the placenta, which produces hormones to support the pregnancy, is expelled from the body. This leads to a rapid decrease in pregnancy hormones, including estrogen and progesterone.

Thyroid hormones, which play a vital role in regulating metabolism and energy levels, can fluctuate after childbirth. Some women may experience temporary thyroid imbalances, leading to conditions like postpartum thyroiditis. This is the inflammation of the thyroid after giving birth, and can lead to hyperthyroidism initially before progressing to hypothyroidism.

Cortisol, known as the stress hormone, may increase temporarily after childbirth due to the physical and emotional stress associated with labor, birth, and the postpartum period.

However, oxytocin, or the bonding hormone, increases as your partner cuddles the new baby. This hormone also surges during childbirth, as it helps with uterine contractions. It can also help with milk ejection during breastfeeding.

Prolactin is the hormone responsible for stimulating milk production in the breasts. After childbirth, prolactin levels surge, signaling the body to produce breast milk to nourish the newborn. This hormone can kick in even if your wife doesn't plan to breastfeed (Watson, 2020).

The rapid hormonal changes after childbirth can impact mood and emotions. Many women experience the "baby blues," characterized by mood swings, irritability, and weepiness, which usually resolve within the first two weeks postpartum. In some cases, PPD or anxiety may occur, which require professional support and treatment.

Myths Versus Facts

The previous symptoms are commonly experienced, but not every new mother will go through them. However, there are a lot of myths involved with the postpartum period. In this section, I'll go over some of those that my clients frequently ask about, and share the facts to help you understand what your partner is really going through in this period.

Myth: Women Bounce Back to Their Prepregnancy Body Within Six Weeks

This myth is laughably inaccurate, because not only do bodies not bounce back like that, no one should expect them to! Six weeks is an alarmingly short period of time when you think of it. Now add in healing from childbirth and caring for a newborn—trust me, that time passes in a blink!

While your partner might lose some weight after childbirth and delivering the placenta, and possibly from breastfeeding, they're not exactly ready to hit the gym. Most women aren't even cleared for high-impact workouts until the six-week checkup. If the birth went well, it's possible to complete light exercises a few days after childbirth, but that's basically walking and stretching. Women who go through cesarean sections are restricted even from that, as they need a longer recovery from the incision (McCallum, 2021).

Myth: Cesarean Babies Aren't as Healthy as Those Born Vaginally

While babies born via cesarean don't have exposure to the same bacteria as those who go through a vaginal birth, it's possible to restore this microbiome development after birth (Neu & Rushing, 2011). Therefore, there's nothing that says a baby born by C-section won't be as healthy as one born vaginally. The key here is that you want your baby and partner in the best possible shape, so whatever method of birth is the most effective is the clear choice.

Myth: Postpartum Women Can't Exercise

It's crucial that a new mother rest after giving birth, but her medical provider will advise her about what exercise she can handle. Mothers recovering from a cesarean should take it easier than those who go through a vaginal birth. As long as your partner follows medical advice and listens to her body, stays hydrated, and gets plenty of rest, she can exercise safely a few days after giving birth (McCallum, 2021).

Myth: Breastfeeding Is the Best Way to Feed Your Baby

The phrase "Breast is best" is one you hear so much during pregnancy and postpartum that you just want to scream, even if you do plan to breastfeed your baby. It gets frustrating because it's a black and white statement, and giving birth and raising a baby involves shades of gray you've never even considered. I'll admit that, yes, breast is best—if it's possible! You don't have to worry about packing bottles for a day out. You don't have the expense of formula. Your partner can pump to try and increase their supply, ensuring they have breast milk handy so you can feed the baby, too. And yes, there are plenty of nutritious reasons that breastfeeding is beneficial for your newborn, like giving them the ideal balance of vitamins, fat, and protein to help boost their immune system and lower their risk of asthma and allergies.

But not everyone can breastfeed. Some women can't stand the pain and discomfort. Some women don't produce enough milk. Some babies can't latch. Some women simply don't want to. There's no shame in giving your baby formula, because they'll get the nutrients they need from that approach, too. The most important thing is to ensure your baby gets enough to eat and can digest the breast milk or formula you feed them (Taylor, 2008).

Myth: Postpartum Women Can't Get Pregnant Immediately

If you know the phrase "Breast is best," you probably also know the myth that breastfeeding means your partner can't get pregnant. While breastfeeding can suppress ovulation, it's not an effective method of birth control (de Bellefonds, 2022). Some women don't get periods while breastfeeding, while others do. But basically, your partner can get pregnant before she has her first period after giving birth. That means she can be pregnant as early as four weeks after giving birth!

Even if you're okay with having another baby so close to your current newborn, the Centers for Disease Control and Prevention (CDC) recommends that women wait at least a year before getting pregnant again. Conceiving within 18 months of giving birth increases your chances of having a premature or low-birth-weight baby, which can cause other developmental delays (de Bellefonds, 2022). It's better to assume your partner is always fertile and take steps toward preventing pregnancy until she's fully healed and you've bonded with your baby for a year or 18 months.

Myth: All Women Experience the Baby Blues

Pretty much every pregnancy and parenting guide addresses the baby blues, so it's easy to assume that all new mothers experience it. However, not every mother feels this way. She may get through the postpartum period without many mood disturbances, though mood swings are common as her hormones level out and she adapts to her new role as a mother.

It's also important to address that not everything that looks like baby blues is that innocent. Baby blues and PPD have many overlapping symptoms. That's why I've devoted an entire chapter—the next one—

to mental health and the mood disorders your partner may experience in the fourth trimester. This issue can be serious, so it's crucial you know what to look for and how to support your partner. Let's jump into that now.

In Our Session

If we were having a one-on-one session about your partner's physical health in the postpartum period, I would ask questions about your knowledge of childbirth recovery and get you to think of ways you can help your partner and baby during this time:

- How familiar are you with the physical changes and recovery process that your partner will go through after giving birth?

- Have you and your partner discussed her expectations for postpartum recovery and how you can assist her during this time?

- What are some practical ways you can help your partner manage her physical comfort as she recovers from childbirth?

- How can you contribute to making sure she's resting and getting the nutrition she needs?

- How can you actively participate in caring for the baby to provide your partner with physical relief and rest?

- Are there specific tasks related to baby care that you can take on to give her some time to recover?

Chapter 3:

Mental Health

Jeana was a client I met a few weeks after she and her new son returned home from the hospital, when she started to feel like she was losing a grip on her life. Jeana had a natural birth and was completely flying on the adrenaline rush she felt after bringing her baby into the world without medical intervention. She told me that even her body didn't seem too sore—she legitimately felt good all over! Until the baby blues hit. Her mood swings were something she'd never felt before. She couldn't control them or even think logically through them because she'd always trusted her mind before, and couldn't fathom how it seemed to play tricks on her now. She'd get incredibly angry at herself for forgetting to pump an extra bottle of breast milk and stopped making time to rest or shower because she wanted the house to look great.

These mood swings, depressive instances, and manic periods went beyond the baby blues, but Jeana couldn't see that, and her partner was working overtime to meet a deadline. One night she had enough. The baby was crying and Jeana could smell her own body odor because she'd gone so long without bathing. She was running on no sleep and thought her nerves were frazzled, but it was more than that. She called her husband and begged him to come home because her son was in distress. Thankfully, her partner heard something in Jeana's voice and raced home. He packed up his wife and the baby and went to the hospital to get help for Jeana. After medication calmed her down, Jeana and her doctor figured out a treatment plan with a psychiatrist and counselor to help her get through PPD.

Sally, on the other hand, was sure she'd experience PPD because she had felt anxious during her entire pregnancy. She worried that she wouldn't be a good mother. She fretted that she had bought the wrong car seat, and could envision the stroller collapsing when she took her baby out for a walk. She was so stressed that she knew the hormone fluctuation and baby blues would progress into full-blown depression after childbirth. However, once the baby was born, Sally held him in her arms and felt all those worries leave her. She couldn't look into his sweet little face and worry about things, because she was consumed with love. That shaped her feelings into a positive mindset that helped her appreciate every moment with her baby, even when he peed onto her shoulder during a diaper change! While many women experience mood issues because of the stress of new motherhood and their hormone levels changing rapidly, not every woman will go through this, so you shouldn't pre-emptively worry.

Though Jeana had never experienced any mental health issues, she still had PPD. However, if your partner has a prior history of depression, anxiety, or other mental health conditions, they're at an elevated risk of experiencing PPD. They can confide in you and their medical provider to ensure someone is always looking out for their well-being, as these symptoms can come on quickly and really make your partner risk their life, as well as your newborn's.

Postpartum mental health is an important topic to address, yet many people don't want to talk about it. Sweeping it under the rug shames women who experience this mood disorder. They feel like, if they were a better mother, they wouldn't feel this way. In reality, PPD isn't something you can just will away, especially if you have a history of mental health issues. On top of experiencing an array of emotions as you adapt to postpartum life, you're also adjusting to being a mother and putting someone else first, which can make you feel out of sorts.

What many people don't realize is that partners are also affected by PPD. One in ten new fathers struggles with anxiety and PPD (Horsager-Boehrer, 2021). Men can experience declining testosterone during their partner's pregnancy and fourth trimester, which impacts their mental health. It can also feel alienating to see your partner bond with the baby so deeply while you don't have as much of a connection with them. You feel lonely because both of the other people in your household are consumed with each other, and you're left on the fringes. On top of that, you're often the one keeping things together. You can go back to work without worrying about pumping. You're doing more household chores as your partner heals. However, you're still taking care of the baby and losing sleep at night, but many people overlook the father's role at this early stage. You can feel alone and unappreciated, which will greatly impact your moods and mental health.

Recognizing and treating any signs of mood disorders is crucial during the fourth trimester, but you also want to stay aware of this type of issue until your baby is older, as it can sneak up on you in times of stress. While society may try to keep this condition in the dark, especially in men, open communication with your partner and medical professionals can significantly help you both—plus your new baby. There's no reason for you or your partner to suffer in silence. Read on to learn more about the various mood disorders you and your partner may experience on the parenthood journey and how you can prioritize and foster positive mental health in the process (Jones et al., 2010).

Perinatal Mood Disorders

Perinatal mood disorders are a group of conditions that can affect women during pregnancy and the postpartum period, and can include emotional and psychological challenges. The most common include PPD, postpartum anxiety, and postpartum PTSD. While exact causes aren't known, all these conditions are treatable with medication, support groups, and lifestyle adjustments (Kerr, 2023).

Common perinatal mood disorders include the following

- perinatal depression

- postpartum anxiety

- postpartum PTSD

- postpartum OCD

- postpartum psychosis

Perinatal mood disorders can impact any woman, regardless of her background or medical history. However, some risk factors increase the likelihood that your partner will experience these conditions. Family mental health history is a major indicator of what may happen during pregnancy and after giving birth. Women who have previously experienced perinatal mood disorders during another pregnancy are also more likely to go through them again. Women with a history of trauma, abuse, financial stress, and a lack of social support are also more likely to experience these conditions. Having pregnancy complications or going through trauma during childbirth also increases the likelihood of perinatal mood disorders.

It's crucial for you and your partner to know the signs of perinatal mood disorders as early detection can make a huge difference to the outcome. You should do all you can to ensure your partner receives the care and compassion needed during this vulnerable time.

Perinatal Depression

PPD is the most well-known mood disorder women experience after giving birth. However, many women are surprised that they can have depression during pregnancy, too. This is called prenatal depression. It often happens due to a combination of hormonal, emotional, and physical factors, along with changing hormones and external factors depending on their support system and life circumstances. Pregnant women often worry about the baby, their body, and how their life will change, so it's understandable that prenatal depression can develop. Prenatal depression can be mild, moderate, or severe (Wisner, 2022).

One of the most precarious issues involving prenatal depression is that it's not only detrimental to the mother's well-being, but can also impact her relationship with the baby. She might have trouble bonding or feel too anxious about the baby to take care of herself. Besides the mother's health, there's a potential for harm to come to the baby as well. Babies born to mothers who experience prenatal depression may have an increased risk of developmental and behavioral issues. If prenatal depression goes untreated, it can worsen into PPD after giving birth.

While the baby blues are a common, temporary emotional state that many mothers experience after giving birth, it's not as severe as PPD. Baby blues are relatively mild, with mood swings, crying spells, irritability, and anxiety happening as a result of hormonal changes and sleep deprivation. As a woman's body adjusts to new motherhood, typically within two weeks, the baby blues ease away. There's no need for medical intervention.

However, women with PPD experience these symptoms more intensely, and they don't ease up. They're persistent and can worsen over time. While baby blues don't require professional intervention, PPD definitely does, and early detection is beneficial for lessening the harmful effects of this condition (Ross et al., 2005).

Women with PPD may experience prolonged periods of sadness and helplessness. They may feel worthless and empty. They don't enjoy activities that used to bring them joy. Some mothers can't even bond with their new baby during this time because they don't see the point.

A new baby in your life will impact your sleep patterns, appetite, and energy. PPD compounds these factors even more, so mothers feel like there's no reason to do anything, including sleep, eat, and shower (Pietrangelo, 2022).

PPD doesn't have a specific cause, but medical professionals note that there are genetic factors that can play a role. That means if women in your partner's family have experienced PPD, she is more likely to have it, too. She also has an increased risk if she has previous diagnoses of mental disorders, or ever went through untreated depressive episodes. Hormonal changes also play a big part in PPD, along with other stressors.

Regardless of the cause, PPD is treatable with medication and counseling. Your partner can talk to psychiatrists and therapists for help managing their symptoms and overcoming this condition. Recognizing the signs is the best way to get a jump on treatment. As soon as you see these symptoms in your partner, ensure they feel supported and get help to protect your family. Discussing PPD and treating it without shame is the best way to raise awareness and reduce the stigma so all new mothers feel empowered to get the help they need.

Postpartum Anxiety

Postpartum anxiety is a common mood disorder that people often overlook. Many people experience anxiety in different areas of their lives, such as social anxiety. Therefore, feeling anxious as a new parent is incredibly understandable. However, postpartum anxiety is more severe. It's a persistent worry that can disrupt the new mother's daily life (Nakić Radoš et al., 2018).

There are many symptoms of postpartum anxiety that go hand in hand with baby blues and PPD, so keep a close eye on your partner to see how severe their issues may be. For example, new parents can experience constant worry. Bringing a baby into the world and knowing you can't protect them forever is enough to make you fret, but the worries of postpartum anxiety are more irrational than that. A new parent may obsessively check on the baby even if they've just put them to bed. They may not be able to relax or sleep because they worry something will happen to the baby. Many new parents with postpartum anxiety are restless because they feel agitated and can't sit still. If they do fall asleep, they have trouble staying asleep because they're on high alert, listening for something to go wrong from the baby's crib (Collier, 2021).

Physical symptoms of anxiety can also present, such as a racing heart, shaky hands and extremities, sweating, feeling dizzy, or being unable to catch your breath. Postpartum anxiety can cause intrusive thoughts, such as the mother harming herself or the baby. These thoughts are alarming because the mother would never follow through and doesn't desire to harm anyone, but the thoughts appear in her mind and make her feel even more anxious (Jondle, 2019).

Some new parents experiencing postpartum anxiety go through avoidance. They avoid people, places, and situations that they worry will put their baby at risk. For example, a new mother may worry about her baby getting sick and dying, so she avoids taking her baby into crowded stores. She might worry about a car jumping the curb and crushing the stroller, so she avoids taking the baby on walks. She may worry about a stranger picking up her baby to hold and running off, so she avoids people and keeps her baby close. While being cautious and aware of her surroundings is a proactive way to stay safe, this level of awareness shouldn't negatively impact how the mother acts. Avoidance with postpartum anxiety can limit daily activities and social interactions, pushing a mother away from people and hobbies and making her feel more alienated and depressed.

Many factors can contribute to postpartum anxiety, like hormone fluctuation, sleep deprivation, stress, and a history of anxiety and mental issues. While these symptoms may initially seem like standard anxiety, keep an eye on them to suggest treatment and support your partner in any way possible to improve her well-being and ability to bond with the baby.

Treatment can include counseling and support groups. In most cases, it's best to talk about the anxiety to find the root problem and help the mother realize why her worries are irrational. However, it's also possible to take medication to ease the side effects of anxiety. Supporting your partner in this situation will help her feel empowered to take action and navigate through this anxiety.

Postpartum Post-Traumatic Stress Disorder

Postpartum PTSD is characterized by re-experiencing traumatic events from childbirth or postpartum and happens to about 9% of new mothers (Postpartum Post-Traumatic Stress Disorder, 2014). This condition can cause significant mental and emotional distress, to the degree of strongly impairing the new mother's daily life. Postpartum PTSD has symptoms similar to traditional PTSD, and it differs from PPD because it's not solely related to feelings of sadness and hopelessness.

Instead, postpartum PTSD involves symptoms like intrusive memories or flashbacks. These can involve re-experiencing the trauma of childbirth. Some women have nightmares about their birth experience or things they worry could have gone wrong in the process. They can't get over the experience and feel stuck in the moment, reliving the pain without relief.

There are also avoidance symptoms, which means new mothers avoid anything that reminds them of that negative experience. They may try to stay away from hospitals and doctors. They're at risk of further emotional damage because they don't want to talk about their experience and process it, even with the support of you, a therapist, or a medical professional. They want to sweep it under the rug even though it constantly pops up in their thoughts.

Another avoidance symptom is hating the idea of having another child. New mothers with postpartum PTSD resist this idea, or even avoid the conversation, because they don't want to risk going through that traumatic experience again.

The other symptom classification is reactive. These symptoms involve heightened anxiety in reaction to certain events. For example, a new mother may be hypervigilant about things happening around her baby because she's overly aware of things that may go wrong. Because her body and mind are always active and on edge, she may have issues sleeping. Without rest, she won't have time to heal physically or emotionally. Lack of sleep can also mean she has trouble concentrating and make her feel irritable during the day (Schwab et al., 2012).

The symptoms of postpartum PTSD can cause persistent feelings of fear and anxiety, sometimes leading to panic attacks. The mother can have trouble sleeping because her anxiety is on such high alert, it won't let her mind or body relax enough to get rest. Over time, these feelings compound so that she feels detached from real life. This can make it tough for her to bond with the baby or even feel emotionally connected with other loved ones.

Postpartum PTSD isn't solely an outcome of mental health issues, like PPD is. Instead, it's more likely to happen if the mother has a difficult childbirth experience. This can include complications involving the birth, emergency interventions, or experiencing a life-threatening occurrence while giving birth. It can also happen if she feels like she lost control during the birthing process.

A lack of support or feeling mistreated during birth can also cause PTSD. Women need to feel like their medical providers listen to them, prioritize their feelings, and keep them and their baby safe. If this doesn't happen, the new mother is likely to feel violated and traumatized by the birth experience and is more likely to develop postpartum PTSD.

That said, it's still possible that previous trauma and pre-existing mental health conditions can lead to postpartum PTSD. Women who went through abuse or sexual assault may feel more vulnerable to having a traumatic birth experience, which can result in PTSD because the situation triggers their memories. Women with a history of anxiety or depression are also more susceptible to develop postpartum PTSD based on their mental well-being.

Treatment for postpartum PTSD is crucial to ensure the new mother is able to come to terms with her past experiences, move on in a healthy way to adjust to motherhood, and feel empowered to open up to her baby and loved ones completely, without fear.

Postpartum Obsessive-Compulsive Disorder

Postpartum OCD is a type of OCD that occurs within the first few weeks after childbirth. Studies have shown that about 11% of new moms screen as positive for postpartum OCD two weeks after giving birth (Miller et al., 2013). By six months postpartum, about half of those mothers still had OCD markers, while other mothers had developed new symptoms. With that in mind, it's crucial to know the signs and get help for your partner so they can manage their transition into motherhood.

Postpartum OCD differs from PPD, postpartum anxiety, and PTSD because it takes the hallmarks of OCD and applies them to the mother's newborn. This means she's more likely to have intrusive, distressing thoughts that inspire and encourage repetitive behaviors (Hudak & Wisner, 2012). The unwanted thoughts are the obsessive aspect, and the repetitive actions are the compulsions.

Symptoms of postpartum OCD vary depending on the mother and her situation, but they always focus on thoughts of harming the baby and doubts about being a good parent, and result in intolerable anxiety. The compulsions are repetitive acts the mother does to try and reduce the anxiety caused by the obsessions (Geddes, 2021). For example, a mother may worry about her baby getting sick, so she washes her hands more often than necessary. She may fear getting stuck away from home without a bottle or diapers, so she checks the diaper bag compulsively, even though she just checked five minutes ago and knows she has everything she needs.

Women with postpartum OCD often feel scared to admit their feelings to anyone else. They worry that people will judge them or label them unfit for motherhood. By supporting your partner and talking openly about the symptoms you notice, you can help remove the stigma from this condition.

Many mothers realize that their compulsions are irrational, but they still can't stop their reactions (Gorbis, 2023). They might initially think the compulsions are harmless. For example, it's better to check the diaper bag for the 10th time instead of realizing you're out of diapers when you're away from home. However, the mental toll these obsessions and compulsions have on a new mother can cause more harm than she initially realizes, and, before long, it becomes too difficult to try and stop the behaviors or change her thinking patterns.

There's no specific known cause of postpartum OCD, but it's most likely a combination of hormones and biological and psychological conditions that contribute to its presence. Hormones and brain chemistry change after childbirth, which can trigger the symptoms. However, when you consider the stress of protecting and raising a newborn, it's understandable that some new mothers can't keep their fears and worries in check.

Regardless of the cause, keeping the symptoms manageable and starting treatment as early as possible will keep the obsessions and compulsions from becoming too severe for the mother to handle. Therapy, medication, support groups, and care from her partner and family will greatly help new mothers manage this condition.

Postpartum Psychosis

Postpartum psychosis is a rare condition that occurs as a result of one or two births in every 1,000, or about 0.1–0.2% (Postpartum Psychosis, 2014). Because it's so rare, many people only hear about it when it's in the news, such as the recent example of a mother experiencing hallucinations before killing her three children (Chuck & McShane, 2023). This condition isn't talked about enough to remove the stigma, so situations like that happen due to lack of treatment and support. The condition is a medical emergency because it has a rapid onset and can escalate quickly, posing a major risk to mother and baby.

It's possible to see symptoms of postpartum psychosis as early as two weeks after childbirth, but it can appear months after the birth (Slivinski, 2022). Symptoms vary, but they are severe and may include hallucinations, delusions, and extreme mood swings. Hallucinations can be visual or auditory, meaning women may see and hear things that aren't there. Delusions are beliefs not rooted in reality, like thinking the baby is possessed and will harm the mother or others if left to their own devices. Mothers experiencing delusions may feel like they're being watched or will be harmed. While mood swings are common during pregnancy and the fourth trimester, postpartum psychosis involves extreme mood swings that can take a new mother from euphoria to agitation in seconds.

Other symptoms include disorganized thoughts and issues with communication. Women with postpartum psychosis are incapable of focusing on their thoughts enough to share them with others. They can also feel confused and disoriented, which may make them have issues facing reality and reacting to their surroundings (Raza & Raza, 2022).

Postpartum psychosis can include hyperactivity, like manic energy levels, or agitation and restlessness. Many women experiencing postpartum psychosis can't sleep due to insomnia. If they manage to fall asleep, they often have a disruption that wakes them up and makes it tough for them to get back to sleep.

The causes of postpartum psychosis are unknown, but most likely include a mix of biological, psychosocial, genetic, and hormonal factors. As with other postpartum disorders, family history plays a part in this condition. Women who are bipolar or had postpartum psychosis with previous births are at a higher risk for this condition. However, it's also possible that the postpartum period contributes to this issue with the lack of sleep for new mothers, paired with hormone fluctuations.

Since postpartum psychosis is a medical emergency, your first reaction should be to call 911 or take your partner to the emergency room. You'll also want to contact their primary doctor. Your immediate goal is to prevent your partner from harming themselves or the baby, so if you're unable to take them to the hospital immediately, remove access to harmful objects like sharp items or medication. Don't leave your partner alone; support them and let them know you're there for whatever they need.

Even after your partner receives medical treatment, you'll want to stay available for them and the baby. Educate yourself about the condition and their treatment options so you can help. Follow all medical advice from the hospital and doctor. Continue to check in with medical professionals and mental health services as recommended. However, know that women can recover from this condition and go on to live fulfilling lives and be amazing mothers and partners. As with other conditions, early intervention is key, and your support is crucial for your partner's well-being.

Treatment Options

Perinatal mood disorder treatment varies depending on the condition and the severity of the issue. These options won't apply to every woman or every disorder, but they are suggestions for starting points you can discuss with your partner and medical team to see what might best help resolve the issue.

Most common is psychotherapy. Therapy options include counseling, cognitive behavioral therapy (CBT), and interpersonal therapy. Talking through issues can greatly help new mothers realize which thoughts are real and logical and which are baseless worries. CBT is a type of therapy that focuses on identifying and changing negative thought processes that cause psychological distress. As negative thoughts can lead to unhealthy behaviors, getting to the root of the issue can make a huge difference in the life and mindset of a new mother. Interpersonal therapy is a short-term approach to therapy that focuses on boosting interpersonal relationships so the new mother feels more supported and knows how to ask for help to improve her emotional well-being.

Medication is another option, either on its own or in partnership with psychotherapy. Medical professionals can prescribe antidepressants or anti-anxiety medication that will alleviate symptoms and help the mother feel more grounded in reality and calm. There are medication options that are healthy to take during pregnancy and breastfeeding, so don't hesitate to get support for your partner during those times.

Support groups can help, in conjunction with the two previous methods or perhaps on their own, depending on the disorder and its severity. Sometimes new mothers feel alone and alienated because their lives have completely changed. They have gone through pregnancy and childbirth, so their bodies may feel unfamiliar. They need to provide constant care to a newborn but also should prioritize their health and recovery, so they often feel pulled in many directions at once. Talking with other mothers can help them feel less alone. They'll hear that other women experience similar thoughts and feelings, so they won't think they're a terrible mother and worry that they'll never adapt to this life change. Support groups are a great source of validation and coping strategies for new parents.

Education about the various mood disorders, such as the previous sections in this chapter, is an important way to help new parents understand what's going on and how to react to their changing circumstances. People unaware of these mood disorders might feel unmoored and worry that they're unable to cope with parenthood, which can lead to negative behaviors and rash decisions. Therefore, being educated about the possibilities is crucial to empower you and your partner to make it through this phase of life in a healthy manner.

Family support is also crucial, which you already know as a partner who sought out this book! As previously mentioned, mothers often feel incredibly alone after giving birth. It's true that new fathers are also struggling to adapt to life with a newborn, but mothers, who are also physically and emotionally healing, feel even more alienated during this time. Support is the best way to keep your partner rooted in reality. Help around the house, spend time caring for your baby, and give your partner plenty of time to rest and recuperate. Keep an eye out for the symptoms of perinatal mood disorders so you can get help as soon as you notice an issue. Your partner will most likely feel so overwhelmed during the fourth trimester that she won't notice if her behaviors and actions are off because she's too close to the issue. Your role during this time is to support and help her in every way possible. Along with your support, ensure that there's no judgment. You don't want your partner to feel ashamed of her thoughts and behaviors because it's not how she truly thinks and feels—it's the mental disorder taking over.

Postpartum Issues in New Fathers

Postpartum mental health is not limited to mothers; it also applies to fathers. The period after childbirth, or the fourth trimester, can be an emotionally challenging time for both parents. Many people don't talk about what fathers go through after childbirth, which is fair because their body didn't give birth to a baby and need extensive recovery. However, fathers can experience emotional and mental impacts from having a baby, so you shouldn't overlook or dismiss anything you're going through as a new parent.

While PPD is more commonly associated with mothers, research has shown that fathers can also experience PPD. Paternal PPD may manifest in symptoms such as feelings of sadness, irritability, fatigue, changes in appetite, difficulty sleeping, and a sense of detachment from the baby. Keep an eye on your symptoms just as you look over your partner's well-being. Your symptoms may be similar to what mothers go through, or they may be different. If you have a history of depression or other mental health issues, you may be more likely to experience PPD.

Becoming a new parent is a major life transition that can be both joyful and overwhelming. Dads may need time to adjust to their new role and responsibilities as a father, which can impact their mental well-being.

Many people give support and attention to mothers because they're in the spotlight with the new baby, while the father is seen more as a secondary character. However, you should ensure you're taking equal care of the new baby and being involved in bonding while caring for your partner. You want to work hard to develop a strong connection with your newborn, as this can help you feel more confident in your new role.

The demands of caring for a newborn can result in sleep deprivation for both parents. Lack of sleep can contribute to mood changes and increased stress. Dads should prioritize rest and seek help from family or friends to share the responsibilities of childcare. This is especially crucial if you don't have parental leave or intend to work as you adapt to life with your new baby. Your wife needs sleep to help her body heal from childbirth and to get rest after caring for the baby, but you also need sleep to ensure you can do your best at work every day. Taking shifts may be the best way to guarantee you can each get several consecutive hours of sleep or even a few full nights' sleep each week.

Engaging actively in parenting activities can strengthen the bond between fathers and their babies. Being involved in caregiving, playing, and spending quality time with the baby can enhance the father–child relationship and promote positive mental health. You can balance that by engaging in stress-relieving activities, such as exercise, hobbies, or spending time with friends. This can help dads manage their emotional well-being during the postpartum period (Horsager-Boehrer, 2021).

Open communication and support between partners are crucial during the postpartum period. Dads should feel comfortable expressing their emotions and concerns about parenthood. Sharing feelings with their partner or seeking support from friends, family, or a mental health professional can be beneficial.

Dads should be aware of signs of distress in themselves and their partners. If you notice symptoms of PPD or anxiety in either yourself or your partner, it's essential to seek professional help promptly. Feelings of sadness, anxiety, or distress can persist or become overwhelming. In that case, dads shouldn't hesitate to get support from a mental health professional. Talking to a therapist or counselor can provide valuable guidance and coping strategies.

It's important to emphasize that experiencing these emotions doesn't make you any less capable or loving as a father. Just as it's normal for mothers to feel the baby blues or PPD, fathers can also go through a similar type of emotional turbulence. Acknowledging these emotions is the first step toward understanding and managing them effectively.

Postpartum issues for fathers are normal and should not be stigmatized. The emotional journey of becoming a father is as significant as that of becoming a mother. The key is to recognize that emotions are a natural response to the enormous changes occurring in your life. While feeling down, upset, or even angry is okay, it's essential to manage these emotions in a healthy way. These feelings can easily get out of hand when you add in the major life transition, lack of sleep, and other complications you feel pressuring you at this important time. By communicating openly, seeking support, practicing self-care, and reaching out for professional help if needed, fathers can navigate the postpartum period with resilience and strength, ultimately contributing positively to their own well-being and that of their growing family.

Recognizing that fathers, like mothers, can experience a range of emotions during the postpartum period is a way to highlight an issue that is often glossed over. The key is to be aware of your mental well-being, seek support when needed, and maintain open communication with your partner and health-care providers. Providing a supportive and understanding environment for both parents can promote positive mental health during this significant life transition.

In Our Session

If we were having a one-on-one session about mental health during the postpartum period, I would ask you some of the following questions to see how you're holding up:

- Are you aware of common mental health concerns that can arise in the postpartum period, such as PPD or postpartum anxiety? How informed are you about the signs and symptoms?

- How often do you check in with your partner about how she's feeling emotionally? How can you make these conversations a regular part of your routine?

- Have you noticed any situations or factors that seem to trigger stress or anxiety for your partner? How can you work together to minimize those triggers?

- How have you been feeling since becoming a dad? Have you noticed any significant changes in your mood or emotions?

- Have you experienced any feelings of stress, anxiety, or overwhelm? How are you managing those emotions?

- Which aspects of being a new dad have been particularly stressful for you? Are there specific situations or factors that trigger feelings of stress or anxiety?

- What are some of the positive emotions you've been experiencing as a new dad?

- Have you felt comfortable expressing your emotions and seeking support when needed?

Chapter 4:

Becoming New Parents

Julia started maternity leave the day before she went into labor, so she was excited to have six weeks to bond with her baby before going back to work. Her husband's job offered parental leave, so they made grand plans to bond as a family for a month or so before starting to transition back to work. However, Julia's birth didn't go as planned, and the baby blues hit her hard. She moped around for two weeks and couldn't appreciate the time with her family. She sought medical attention to ensure her mood disorder wasn't PPD, but still couldn't shake how dejected she felt. Her husband stepped up to take care of household chores and feed the baby, but that made Julia feel worse because she wasn't bonding with the baby. She realized that her return to work looming over her head made her focus more on the ticking clock than on spending time with her newborn. She and her husband started planning short outings to take the baby around the city, and Julia felt better after leaving the house. She realized that she was actually excited to go back to work, which made her feel guilty because she thought she should feel hesitant to put her baby in daycare. However, once she accepted that she loved her job and her baby would flourish in the small daycare they'd carefully chosen, Julia was able to embrace herself while still bonding with her baby. She shed the idea that she needed to act a certain way to be a good mother and accepted who she was.

Kim was my first client who was becoming a mom for the second time! She had a three-year-old son who stayed at home with his grandmother while Kim and her husband, Kyle, went to the hospital to have their daughter. Though Kim had gone through the fourth trimester before, she had never done it with another child at home, and thought my advice could help her manage this transition. Many people think that adding another baby to the family is no big deal—after all, you've done it before, so what else is new? However, every baby is unique. Women who had an easy pregnancy and birth may experience the exact opposite the second time around. Children also have drastically different personalities. In this case, Kim's son was very active and loved attention. She was worried she wouldn't be able to rest and care for the baby without her son feeling left out. Since her husband had a demanding job in the medical field, I helped Kim make a plan to arrange childcare and playdates and set up things to keep her son occupied while she rested and took care of the newborn. When Kim brought her daughter home from the hospital, the baby gave her big brother a new toy, which immediately endeared him to his baby sis! He always wanted to be around her, but quickly learned that his mom and sister needed to rest. Kim enjoyed having her son bond with her and the new baby, but also made the most of the time he was away or looked after by someone else. She made sure she napped and showered whenever she had the chance so she felt rested and energized enough to mother two children when necessary. Instead of feeling selfish for taking this time for herself, Kim realized it was the best option because she felt great when both kids were around, but was able to move at a slower pace when it was just her and the baby.

Having a baby is a very exciting time in any parent's life, whether they've done it before or not. The anticipation of meeting the new little one, watching them grow, and creating lasting memories is a profound experience. However, amid the excitement, the prospect of bringing a new life into the world can be both thrilling and overwhelming. As you embark on this journey of parenthood, it's essential to understand what it means to become new parents, whether for the first time or again, and equip yourselves with suggestions and strategies to ease the transition for everyone involved.

The bottom line is that you have to embrace the journey. Julia thought motherhood would look peaceful and serene, with her nursing the baby in a rocking chair. But that just wasn't her. She's not the type of person to slow down and change her personality, and that's fine! You are who you are, and your baby will adjust to that. In time, they'll respect you more for it because you've shown them that you can be yourself and adapt to the world around you. You'll also feel better because you're not giving up part of yourself to be what you deem an "ideal" parent. Kim's situation was similar. Though she's a stay-at-home mom, she was worried that sending her older child away for long playdates would make it seem like she couldn't handle two children or wasn't pulling her weight as a stay-at-home parent. However, it was just an adjustment period that required certain actions, not a permanent solution. Embracing the journey and being flexible, especially the first few months postpartum, is a crucial quality for both partners.

Most parenting books focus on pregnancy and labor, then jump ahead to raising a child in terms of routine, discipline, and helping them become productive members of society. However, you need to educate yourself about the postpartum period, as covered in this book. Understanding what will happen as you experience childbirth, bring the baby home, and acclimate to this new lifestyle can greatly prepare you to handle all the obstacles that will come your way. You can talk to other parents with this experience, ask advice from medical professionals, read books, and attend classes that focus on new parenthood. Along with knowing what to expect as a parent, you should also learn about the baby's developmental stages and Wonder Weeks, which can help you know what behavioral changes are coming your way. The more information you have, the better prepared you'll feel. Instead of only knowing one way to feed the baby or put them to sleep, you'll have several options at your fingertips so you can pivot to a new solution instead of feeling frustrated that one way isn't working.

In this stage of new parenthood, your support system is key. Knowing that you can reach out to family and friends for various types of support is the best way to keep yourself in check without feeling overwhelmed by your new life. You can ask for help with chores, like asking a friend to pick up a few items at the store when they do their own shopping. You can ask the new grandparents to spend a few hours with the baby to allow you and your partner some time together—or simply quiet time to rest and relax! It's also nice to know you can call up a friend or family member to ask them something about what you're experiencing with your baby and get advice from someone you trust. Parenting groups are also ideal for this type of advice and support. They're a good way to socialize and make friends with parents in the same stage of life as you. Who knows—maybe you'll make lifelong friends and your babies will bond, too!

Bringing Baby Home

Bringing a newborn baby home is a significant milestone that marks the beginning of an exciting journey for new parents. As you cross the threshold of your familiar home, your hearts brim with excitement, trepidation, and boundless love. Your home, once a sanctuary for just the two of you, now echoes with the sweet coos and gentle cries of your precious bundle of joy. With a mixture of anticipation and apprehension, new parents embark on this adventure, ready to embrace the sleepless nights, tender moments, and profound sense of responsibility that parenthood bestows upon them. As you cradle your little one in your arms, you enter a new chapter of life, one filled with laughter, tears, and unbreakable bonds. The world may appear different through the eyes of a new parent, but the love that envelops this tiny new arrival as you bring them home is nothing short of magical. To ensure this transition goes off without a hitch, consider the tips and advice below for smooth sailing.

Babyproofing

Babyproofing is something you most likely thought about or accomplished during pregnancy, as it fits nicely with the nesting process. While your newborn won't roll or crawl for several months, you want to prepare while you have time instead of realizing that you need to babyproof the house once your child is on the go. It's a crucial process to keep your little one safe, as they'll soon want to explore their surroundings and get to know their new home.

Start as soon as you can. You can babyproof the house even before the baby can move independently, just so you don't forget to do it later. That way you'll know your home is a safe space for them when they're ready to explore. The best way to do this is to get down on your hands and knees and see things from your little one's point of view. You might notice things you wouldn't see from an adult's height.

One of the most important babyproofing steps is to cover electrical outlets. You can get safety plugs to put into the outlet, or cover the entire thing with a special cover. Both effectively prevent your baby from sticking their fingers or other objects into the outlet holes.

Window safety is another crucial concern. You can install window stops or guards to keep your baby from falling out of windows when they start exploring. If you have blinds in your windows, install a cord winder to keep the strings from dangling down. You can also choose cordless blinds to eliminate the risk entirely, as the strings hanging will tempt your baby to grab them and pose a strangulation risk.

Electronic cords are also something you should carefully conceal. You don't want your baby to crawl over to a cord and pull it out of the socket, or pull an electronic device down from its perch. Long cords with slack pose a strangulation risk just like blind cords, so keep everything secure and out of your baby's reach.

Use furniture straps and brackets to attach heavy furniture to the walls. All bookshelves and cabinets should be securely held to the wall. You can also anchor electronics like your TV and stereo so they won't fall over or be easy for the baby to pull off their surface.

If your furniture has sharp corners, you'll want to cover the edges with cushioned guards to prevent the baby from getting hurt if they bump or fall against those items (Geddes, 2022).

Baby gates are a great way to keep your baby from exploring the stairs. Put gates at the top and bottom of your inside stairs. You can also put gates across doorways to keep your baby out of certain rooms. As they get a bit older and can play independently, gates will help because you can leave your child in the playroom but easily hear them and peek in without needing to close a wooden door. Some of my clients have also used baby gates to keep their dogs in areas away from the baby, but note that this only works if your dogs are small and can't jump high. Bigger dogs, energetic dogs, and cats won't be deterred by baby gates!

I always recommend putting a baby gate in the kitchen doorway because otherwise, the baby could get access to utensils, knives, and breakable dishware. However, I also advise new parents to put cabinet and drawer locks in the kitchen and bathroom to prevent the baby from getting access to cleaning solutions, plastic bags, toiletries, and more. In terms of the kitchen, you can also get stove-knob covers to prevent the baby from turning on the stove if the knobs aren't completely out of reach.

In addition to cabinet and drawer locks in the bathroom, you should also add a toilet lock. This can prevent drowning, with the added benefit of making it so your baby can't flush away any valuable belongings! You should also keep medications and toiletries out of reach and locked away in a cabinet or drawer. Though you'll help bathe your baby, and often start doing so in the kitchen sink or a smaller plastic tub, it adds an extra layer of safety to apply a nonslip bath mat in the tub, plus a secure bath mat on the tile outside of the tub (Bykofsky, 2023).

Trash cans are another source of interest for babies. Using a covered trash can will keep them from reaching into the container to explore what you've thrown away. Besides preventing a mess, a trash can with a lid will also keep your baby from ingesting anything harmful you've thrown away.

As your baby starts to explore, you'll realize there are a lot of small items in your home, and they're like magnets for your baby. You might not notice anything, but your baby will zero in on a penny that fell next to the coffee table and grab it. Coins, batteries, knickknacks, paper clips, and other small items are the perfect size for your baby to grasp and shove in their mouth, so you want to take a critical eye to your home and put these items out of reach.

Plants are another aspect of home life that will require some research and protection. Just as some plants, like lilies, cyclamen, and aloe vera, are toxic for your furry friends, some plants will harm your baby if ingested. Since babies are curious and will grab anything and put it in their mouths, you should keep your plants somewhere off-limits to your curious little one. Plants like daffodils, hydrangeas, English ivy, peach lilies, philodendron, and azaleas are highly toxic and can irritate your baby's nose or mouth and cause abdominal pain, vomiting, and diarrhea if consumed (Shatzman, 2023). Keeping plants away from your baby while teaching them to look but not touch will ensure you can keep your child safe from this type of issue in your home and yard.

Babyproofing is an ongoing process because your baby will continually develop new skills and abilities. Regularly re-evaluate your babyproofing measures as your child grows and keep adapting your home to ensure a safe and secure environment for them to explore and thrive in.

Adjusting to a New Lifestyle

Preparation is key when you adjust to any new lifestyle, but when it comes to bringing a baby into the world, that isn't always possible. No one knows how labor will progress or how their baby will act when they all come home. But you can prepare in many areas to lessen the stress of adapting to daily life with a newborn. For example, you can stock up on things you know you'll need, like diapers, wipes, and baby clothes. You can get a stroller, car seat, and crib ahead of time, and set up the baby's room before your partner goes into labor. Having all the supplies organized and on hand will help you feel prepared to an extent, giving you more energy and mental capacity to deal with your baby and be more flexible as you adjust (Divecha, 2016).

Help from friends and family will also provide a smooth transition into parenthood. You don't have to trust someone with your baby, but let them pick up the slack in terms of bringing food or running errands while you stay home with your newborn. If you don't have a support system around, you can hire out a lot of tasks in the first few months. Grocery and food delivery services can be a lifesaver. Splurge on a landscaping crew instead of pushing yourself to mow your own yard. It can cost more, but it's just a short-term investment to give yourselves time to rest and adjust to parenthood, which will serve you well in the long run. Instead of starting from zero and depleting yourselves, you'll bond with your baby and feel more in control of your new life, which puts you in a position of empowerment. As the baby gets older, you can take back some of these chores and errands without feeling even more overwhelmed than you were during the newborn stage.

Even though you can accept help from your support system, don't feel compelled to accept all their advice. As a new parent, you can definitely get information from people who have been there and done that, whether they're friends, family, or experts in the field. But the bottom line to remember is that you should trust your gut and make the choices that seem right to you. So much of parenting is flying by the seat of your pants. Even those parents who seem like they have it all together have doubts, so don't feel like anyone knows better than you. You know yourself and your partner, and you know how you want to raise your child. Trusting your instincts when your baby's a newborn will help you find your footing and become more confident in your parenting abilities (Salazar, 2019).

To trust your gut like that, you need to feel like your best self. That means getting enough rest, either napping when the baby naps or alternating night shifts with your partner. Ensure you're both eating regular meals of healthy food. Taking care of yourself is crucial because it's easy to get caught up in your baby's needs and forget about your own. But you need time to rest and recharge your batteries to be the best possible parent for your baby.

Putting yourself first occasionally isn't selfish because it will put you in a better position to bond with your baby. You won't feel exhausted and overwhelmed, passively holding your baby while you feed them a bottle. You'll have the energy to engage with your newborn by cuddling, talking, and singing with them. This approach will help you strengthen your emotional connection with your child, which will then continue to develop throughout their life.

The most important thing I tell every client to remember is to give yourself grace. When you're responsible for every aspect of a newborn's life, it's easy to be hard on yourself. So many parents beat themselves up for making a small mistake that would naturally happen as you learn along the way. There's no reason to think you're a terrible parent because your baby got a diaper rash or you didn't warm the bottle enough. These things happen and you'll always learn from your mistakes. No one is perfect and every parent faces challenges, so just roll with the punches and keep doing your best. This period of your baby's life is short and sweet, so make time to enjoy it (Lambert, 2009).

How to Learn to Parent

Learning to parent is an extraordinary journey that requires dedication, patience, and a willingness to grow alongside your child. As new parents embark on this life-changing adventure, they enter a world filled with challenges and endless opportunities for personal development. But it's also crucial to make time to experience the wonder of raising a child and attempt to see the world through their eyes. Nurturing a child's physical, emotional, and cognitive growth demands a diverse set of skills and an open heart, as well as a willingness to adapt to the ever-evolving needs of their little one. By embracing the joys and complexities of parenting, individuals can discover the profound joy of watching their child flourish, while also uncovering newfound strength within themselves. From developing a strong bond with their baby to mastering the art of balancing love and discipline, the path to becoming a confident and capable parent is a transformative process that offers boundless rewards. These tips will help you start the parenting journey on the right path.

Creating a Routine

Creating a routine as a new parent is a valuable tool for establishing stability and predictability in both your baby's life and your own. While the early days of parenthood can feel overwhelming and unpredictable, having a consistent daily schedule can provide a sense of structure that benefits both you and your little one. A well-thought-out routine helps babies feel secure and confident, as they come to anticipate what comes next. Moreover, it can significantly contribute to your well-being as a parent by allowing you to plan and manage your time effectively.

In this process of creating a routine, remember to be flexible and adaptable, as babies' needs change as they grow. For example, as your newborn develops, they won't nap as much throughout the day, so you can add playtime and storytime between each rest period (Fletcher, 2023).

Follow these steps to effectively create a routine for your new family.

Start as soon as you can. You may think that a newborn has no sense of time so it's not worth trying to establish a routine, but adapting your schedule to the baby's will greatly help you make the most of your time. You can sleep when the baby sleeps and have plenty of time to bond with them without feeling like you've sapped all your energy. During the first few weeks of your baby's life, your routine will revolve around eating, sleeping, and bonding.

The easiest way to develop a routine is to follow the baby's natural rhythms. You'll see that they get hungry every couple of hours and then want to sleep. When they wake up, they're alert, so you can play and bond. These times will change as your baby gets older, with less naptime and more playtime, so continue to observe their natural cues and establish your routine around them to prevent them from being too sleepy to play or so hungry they throw a tantrum (Dougherty, 2022).

Consistency is the best way to establish routines. You might get off track every so often if you have something special planned, are traveling, or have guests over, but you should stick to your routine as much as possible. Your baby depends on it, and may get fussy and unsettled without it. If you're consistent with wake-up, nap, and bedtimes, you'll have a happy, healthy baby on your hands, which means you'll be happy and healthy as a parent! However, with that said, it will sometimes happen that you can't stick to your routine. Instead of beating yourself up over it, just be flexible and handle changes the best you can. Sometimes it will be due to something you can't avoid, like teething or a growth spurt that makes your baby inconsolable. Do the best you can and adapt the routine to your baby's needs (Bell, 2021).

Although it may take time and adjustments to find the perfect rhythm for your family, the effort is well worth it in the long run. Embrace the joys of parenthood while nurturing a sense of balance and organization through the power of a thoughtfully crafted routine.

Communicating With Your Partner

Chapter 6 goes in-depth on how you can become the best co-parent with your partner, but knowing some tips about communication will help you as you adjust to bringing your baby home. The first few days of parenthood can feel scary and uncertain, or they may pass by in a blissful haze. Regardless of which type you experience, things will change—often! One day may make you feel like a superhero parent, while the next makes you worry that you'll never have it together enough to raise a decent human. These obstacles will cause you to stumble, but if you can effectively communicate with your partner, you'll have the best support system to get through the rough patches and genuinely enjoy being a parent.

Effective communication with your partner as new parents is essential for navigating the joys and challenges of parenthood together. The arrival of a baby can bring about significant changes to your relationship dynamics, and open, honest, and supportive communication can strengthen your bond and make the transition smoother. These foundational tips will help you communicate with your partner as new parents and hold you over until you get to Chapter 6 for even more relationship advice (Eldemire, 2021).

Discuss Parenting Goals

Discussing parenting goals with your partner is a fundamental aspect of effective communication as new parents. Parenting goals are the shared values, principles, and aspirations that guide how you both want to raise and nurture your child. These discussions are essential for aligning your parenting approaches, making joint decisions, and creating a cohesive and supportive environment for your little one. You might talk about this before you get married, before you have children, and during pregnancy, but once you have a baby your views may change. It's easy to expect parenting to be one way, but as you get involved in it, you realize that your ideal isn't realistic, so you need to change your views. Talking with your partner about goals will help you stay on the same page and feel supported in every choice you make (Diamond, 2023).

Some topics you may want to discuss include how you want to raise the baby in terms of chores, discipline, and responsibility. You should be on the same page about your goals for them. You may want your child to be happy no matter what path they take, while your partner envisions them going to college and leading a more traditional life. Talking about your expectations will help you come together as a team to parent your child in the best way for your family.

Share Your Thoughts

Open and honest communication between parents is crucial because you don't want to keep anything inside and let it fester into resentment. You should always feel encouraged to share your thoughts and feelings with your partner, and encourage them to do the same. It helps to be respectful and open-minded, letting them share everything on their mind before jumping in with your own input. Similarly, your partner should let you talk without interruption. When you know you'll have a chance to make yourself heard, you'll feel more encouraged to talk to your partner. While you may want to focus on parenting, you should also ensure you're making time to talk about your interests, feelings, thoughts, and dreams so you and your partner stay connected as a couple as well as in parenthood.

You can also use this approach as a parenting style as your child grows up. It encourages parents to create a safe and supportive environment where children feel comfortable expressing their thoughts, feelings, and ideas without fear of judgment. Sharing your thoughts with your family promotes emotional well-being, encourages healthy self-expression, and nurtures positive couple and parent–child relationships (Nathanson, 2019).

Listen Actively

Listening actively to your partner is an essential skill for effective communication and building a strong and supportive relationship. Active listening involves being fully present, showing genuine interest, and empathizing with your partner's thoughts and feelings. Give them your full attention instead of engaging with the baby, scrolling on your phone, or watching TV. Maintaining eye contact is a great way to show them you're listening.

Don't interrupt your partner when they talk, and don't make judgments on what they're saying. You should listen to everything they have to say and process it before reacting in any way. Otherwise you might react in a negative way that makes them close themselves off from you. Always try to see things from their point of view and show empathy so they know you're trying to understand. You can also paraphrase or summarize what they've shared with you to ensure you understood what they're saying. If what you say doesn't align with what they meant, they can clarify the situation before it causes an argument or miscommunication.

For example, you may listen to your partner tell you she's so tired she can hardly function, and that she needs you to take on more night responsibilities while she catches up on sleep. If you hear that and keep it inside, you might start to remember it as her accusing you of not doing anything around the house or for the baby, and you may start to feel frustrated or resentful. However, after she speaks, you can repeat what she says to ensure that's what she meant. If you interpreted things in a way she didn't intend, this process gives her a chance to clarify what she meant. Maybe she wanted to express how she felt so tired, she wished you could wave a wand to fix everything and then both of you could get plenty of sleep. She may realize that the way she words things isn't conveying her ideal meaning, so she can work on that to prevent this type of issue in the future. This approach will also give you both a chance to calm your tempers and communicate effectively without letting misconceptions cloud the air and harm your parenting relationship.

Even if you don't agree with your partner, part of active listening includes validating their feelings. For example, they may feel like they're doing the bulk of the parenting. You may not agree, but you can accept that they feel this way for a reason. After you hear them out and reflect on the issue, you can then bring up that you feel like you don't have enough time to bond with the baby because you had to go back to work. Your partner will actively listen to your reply, and then you can address the conflict (Eldemire, 2021).

Address Conflicts

In the whirlwind of postpartum adjustments, it's not uncommon for tempers to run short and for conflicts to arise between partners. You should acknowledge that these challenges are a natural part of the process. The exhaustion, stress, and heightened emotions can sometimes lead to misunderstandings and disagreements. Remember, you and your partner are both on a steep learning curve as you adapt to your new roles as parents.

You might be able to find the triggers behind your disagreements. For example, sleepless nights, changes in routines, and added responsibilities can contribute to heightened emotions. When arguments occur, take a step back to understand what triggered the disagreement. Was it a misunderstanding, a miscommunication, or simply the result of built-up stress? Identifying the root cause can help prevent similar conflicts in the future.

Getting to the meat of the issue can feel challenging, especially if you're stressed or sleep deprived during the newborn phase. With that in mind, it's crucial that you and your partner wait to address conflicts until you have the right time and place to really hash it out. You don't want to have this discussion when you're with the baby at the zoo or at a family member's house for dinner. Wait until you can be alone and truly focus on the conversation, with enough time to figure out possible solutions.

While addressing conflicts, stay calm and respectful. One way to do this is to keep your voice low and don't escalate to yelling or scolding. Using "I" statements will also prevent your discussion from escalating into an argument. Instead of accusing your partner of things, you're framing it from your point of view. You can say, "I feel left out because I don't feed the baby," instead of saying, "You spend more time with the baby because you're breastfeeding." This shift in the point of view prevents accusatory language and helps your partner understand things from your point of view.

Active listening comes into play when addressing conflicts. You should also be willing to take responsibility for your actions. If you've made a mistake or reacted badly, own up to it, apologize, and clear the slate instead of deflecting blame or doubling down on a bad move. This can help avoid escalation and encourage you and your partner to find common ground and assess possible solutions.

Some solutions will involve compromises, so you should both be open to that. It's not always possible that you'll get your way or be proven right in a conflict, and that shouldn't be your goal. As parents, you and your partner have a common purpose that should be your focus now. So, regardless of how you resolve the conflict, you should always end by reaffirming your love for each other and your commitment to the relationship and family. Hearing this will remind you both how much you love each other and why you wanted to marry and start a family. This type of healthy conflict resolution will get easier over time and can reinforce your parenting goals, so it's worth the time and effort to work on this process until it feels natural with your partner (Nathanson, 2019).

Be Patient

Being patient with your partner is essential for maintaining a healthy and harmonious relationship. Patience allows you to understand and support your partner during challenging times and fosters a sense of empathy and understanding.

Patience starts from within. Be aware of your own emotions and triggers. Understanding your feelings can help you manage them better and respond to your partner with patience. When you feel yourself becoming impatient, take deep breaths to calm yourself. This simple technique can help you stay composed during difficult moments.

When you feel in control of yourself, try to see things from your partner's perspective and empathize with their emotions. Empathy allows you to be more understanding and patient with their experiences. Resist making assumptions about your partner's intentions or feelings. Instead, ask for clarification and seek to understand their perspective fully.

When conflicts arise, focus on finding solutions together rather than dwelling on the problem. Work as a team to address challenges. Pay attention to your tone of voice when communicating with your partner. Speaking in a gentle and understanding tone can prevent misunderstandings and defensiveness.

Sometimes, your partner may need space and time to process their emotions. Respect their need for space and avoid pressuring them to talk immediately.

Focus on the positive aspects of your partner and the relationship. Express gratitude for the qualities you appreciate in them. Understand that nobody is perfect and everyone has their strengths and weaknesses. Set realistic expectations for your partner and the relationship.

Remind yourself of your love for and commitment to your partner. This can serve as a reminder to be patient and supportive during challenging times. Being patient with your partner also requires being patient with yourself. Don't be too hard on yourself if you find it challenging at times; instead, practice self-compassion and self-care.

Remember that patience is a virtue that requires practice and effort. By being patient with your partner, you create an atmosphere of trust and support in the relationship, fostering a deeper connection and mutual understanding (Diamond, 2023).

Split Responsibilities

Splitting responsibilities with your partner is essential for creating a balanced and supportive home environment. Effective division of tasks allows both partners to share the workload, reduce stress, and strengthen their partnership in parenting and household duties.

Start by having an open and honest conversation about how you both envision splitting responsibilities. Discuss your strengths, preferences, and areas where you might need more support. Recognize each other's strengths and interests. Assign tasks that align with each partner's skills and abilities. This way, you can both contribute effectively.

Create a list of all the tasks that need to be done regularly, such as childcare, cooking, cleaning, shopping, and paying bills. Divide these tasks between you and your partner based on your preferences and availability. Be open to adjusting the division of responsibilities as needed. Life circumstances may change, so flexibility is essential in adapting to new situations.

Both partners should actively participate in parenting duties, including childcare, bedtime routines, and, eventually, school activities. Share the load of caregiving to bond with your child and support each other.

Set realistic expectations for each other and the tasks at hand. Understand that both of you are human and may have limitations or busy periods. Periodically check in with each other to assess how the division of responsibilities is working. Discuss any adjustments needed to ensure a fair distribution of tasks.

Allow your partner to complete their assigned tasks in their own way and time. Avoid micromanaging or constantly critiquing how they handle their responsibilities. Offer help and support to your partner when needed, even if it's not your designated task. Being a team means being there for each other.

Ensure that both you and your partner have time for self-care and personal pursuits. Taking care of yourselves will make you more effective in handling responsibilities. Involve each other in making important decisions related to family, finances, and household matters. Being part of the decision-making process ensures both partners have a say. Acknowledge and appreciate each other's contributions regularly. Showing gratitude for the efforts made creates a positive and supportive atmosphere.

Remember, the key to successfully splitting responsibilities with your partner is collaboration, communication, and mutual respect. By working as a team and supporting each other, you can create a balanced and loving home environment for your family (Waychoff, 2020).

I've helped a few couples with this by writing chore charts on whiteboards or lists hung in a common area, like the kitchen. I recommend that you get a whiteboard, even if it's a small one that is attached to your fridge with magnets, and write the necessary chores in a list. If they need to be done daily, you can create a calendar grid with blank spaces next to the chore like a checklist. If they have a specific deadline, write that in a bright red marker so it's obvious. As someone completes a chore, they can sign off on the whiteboard using their initials instead of a simple check. After a few weeks of this process, parents start to come together to work as a team and tackle tasks. Using your initials instead of a checkmark can help you both see how much work you're doing. Sometimes people resent their partner deep down because they feel like they're picking up the slack while their partner kicks back. But seeing how much you each do levels the playing field and offers a degree of honest transparency. However, it's also possible that this will truly show how much work one partner is doing compared to the other! In that case, you can assess the chore chart and come up with a way to better split the workload so no one person gets overtaxed and everyone helps out to the best of their abilities.

Schedule Time Together

Scheduling time together with your partner is essential for nurturing your relationship and maintaining a strong emotional bond. Despite busy schedules and other commitments, making intentional efforts to spend quality time together is crucial for the health of your partnership. Look at both of your schedules and find a time that works for both of you. It could be a weekly date night or a set time during the weekend when you can be together without interruptions. Make spending time together a priority. Block off time in your calendars and treat it as an important commitment that you both value. However, remember that life can be unpredictable, so be flexible with your plans. If something comes up and you can't stick to your scheduled time, find another suitable time to be together.

Use your scheduled time to try new activities or experiences together. Exploring new things can add excitement and novelty to your relationship. During your scheduled time together, minimize distractions like phones or work-related matters. Focus on each other and be fully present in the moment.

Be protective of your scheduled time together. Communicate with others, such as family or friends, about the importance of this time for your relationship. Take turns planning activities or outings for your scheduled time together. This way, both partners get a chance to surprise and delight each other. Spending time together doesn't always require elaborate plans. Even simple activities like cooking together, going for a walk, or having a movie night can be meaningful. Make spending time together a regular habit, so it becomes an integral part of your relationship.

Remember that spending time together is an investment in your relationship. It allows you to connect, communicate, and grow as a couple. By making the effort to schedule and prioritize this time, you create a strong foundation for a loving and lasting partnership (Fletcher, 2022).

What Does Parenting Look Like?

Parenting looks different based on the individual's goals for their child, their baby's demeanor, and the source of the parenting advice. For example, many parenting books are fairly strict in their approach, making you feel like you must do exactly as they recommend or else you're failing your child. Then you may look at social media and feel like you need to be going above and beyond for your child, making every day magical and fun, which can be exciting but quickly drains you. Photos and videos shared on social media and parenting blogs are often performative, so you shouldn't consider them an accurate barometer for how you should parent your child. Instead, find one source of advice you can rely on and stick with it. I always recommend my clients talk to their pediatrician and use that information as their basic guidelines. Then they can take in any other advice and weigh it against what they know from their trusted medical professional before deciding if it's worth following or not.

Please note that I include my advice in this section! While I have experience as a parent, along with years of research and coaching under my belt, I'm not an expert compared to your pediatrician. Also, the advice you get from my book is much more generalized than how I can help clients one on one, so it's still something you need to weigh against your thoughts and ideal approach to parenthood. My purpose here is to give you broad ideas of how to parent and adjust to the postpartum period; you can take what's helpful from the book and apply it to your life as needed. I try to give you as much information as possible so you have an idea of how things may go and how to have tools in your kit to help you roll with the punches if things don't go exactly according to plan.

The bottom line of parenting is that it includes unconditional love. You'll experience a deep and unconditional love for your child, unlike anything you've ever felt before. This love will be the foundation of your relationship with your child. Everything you do for your baby comes from a place of love, which can simplify the decision-making process—you'll learn how to trust your gut and see what parenting approach makes you and your baby feel the most love.

However, parenting also requires a lot of sacrifice. You're responsible for a newborn, and you'll have that responsibility for at least the next 18 years, though I'm here to tell you that the worry you'll feel for your child, and the way you'll want to provide for them the best you possibly can, never really goes away. So you're going to make a lot of sacrifices over the years. You'll need to prioritize your child's needs over your own at times, making sure they are safe, healthy, and happy. You're responsible for nurturing your child's physical, emotional, and mental well-being. This involves feeding, bathing, providing a safe environment, and offering emotional support (Curtis-Mahoney & Reilly, 2022).

Parenting can be challenging, and it's normal to face difficult situations. Patience is key during these times, as children may test boundaries and have tantrums. Just like your child, you'll also be on a learning journey. You'll learn about your child's developmental stages, their unique personality, and how to best support their growth. Spend quality time with your child to create memories and build a strong connection. Engage in activities you both enjoy, and be present in their lives. Children often learn by observing their parents. Model the behavior you want to see in your child, such as kindness, respect, and empathy. Celebrate your child's achievements and milestones, no matter how small. It boosts their confidence and shows them that you are proud of them.

Establishing consistent boundaries and discipline is important. Find a balance between being firm and nurturing while setting appropriate limits for your child's behavior. As your child grows, communication becomes crucial. Listen to your child, even when they are young, as it helps build trust and strengthens your bond (Klass & Damour, 2019).

More than anything else, remember to cherish the special moments and enjoy the journey of parenthood. Children grow up quickly, so make the most of each stage.

Flexibility and Adaptation

Becoming a new parent is a life-altering experience that brings immense joy and fulfillment. However, it also comes with a multitude of challenges that require adaptability and flexibility. As you embark on this new stage of life, being open to change and adjusting to the unpredictable nature of parenting can make all the difference in creating a positive and nurturing environment for your child. Parenting rarely goes exactly as planned. Being flexible and adaptable will help you navigate the unexpected twists and turns that come with raising a child.

Parenthood is a dynamic and ever-changing role. As your child grows and develops, their needs, behaviors, and preferences will evolve. Flexibility as a parent means being open to these changes and being willing to adapt your approach accordingly. With the arrival of a child, your priorities will naturally shift. Adaptation involves recognizing that some things may take a backseat temporarily while you focus on your child's well-being. Your social life may change as you focus on your child's needs. Being flexible with your social commitments and finding ways to stay connected with friends and loved ones can help maintain a support system. When you're parenting with a partner, being flexible and willing to share responsibilities is vital. As each of you learns and grows as parents, it's important to adapt together and support one another (Curtis-Mahoney & Reilly, 2022).

For first-time parents, the transition to parenthood can be overwhelming. Flexibility in this phase means recognizing that adjustments take time and seeking support when needed. Newborns and infants have irregular sleep patterns, which can be exhausting for parents. Being flexible with your own sleep schedule and finding ways to rest when possible can help you cope with the demands of caring for a baby (Fletcher & Craft, 2022).

Babies communicate through cries, facial expressions, and body language. Learning to interpret and respond to your baby's cues is crucial for meeting their needs promptly. Being flexible in your routines and attentive to your child's signals fosters a sense of security and trust. As your child grows, they will develop their own personality and interests. Being adaptable as a parent means embracing their individuality and providing support for their unique passions.

For working parents, finding a balance between career and family life requires flexibility. It may involve adjusting work hours, seeking flexible work arrangements, or arranging childcare. Parenting often involves solving various challenges. Flexibility enables you to approach problems with creativity and openness, finding solutions that work best for your family (Klass & Damour, 2019).

Parenthood may not always align with the idealized vision you had before becoming a parent. Flexibility helps in managing expectations and embracing the reality of the journey. No parent is perfect, and there will be moments when you make mistakes or feel uncertain. Flexibility means being forgiving of yourself, learning from challenges, and striving to do better. Parenting is a transformative experience that changes you as a person. Embracing the changes within yourself and your family allows you to grow alongside your child.

Prioritizing Self-Care

You'll learn more about the self-care process in Chapter 5 because it's that important. But, for now, you should know that, without giving yourself some downtime, you'll burn out quickly. Newborns are demanding—they can't do anything for themselves and don't have a routine yet, so you're at their beck and call. If you push yourself to do everything for your baby while still juggling your pre-parent life, you're not going to have the time or energy for everything. You'll work so hard that you eventually won't be able to help with anything, and that's not beneficial for you, your partner, or the baby. Being moderate with your activities and making time for yourself is crucial during the fourth trimester. The best way to do that is to share responsibilities with your partner (Curtis-Mahoney & Reilly, 2022).

These quick tips will help you learn how to add self-care into your daily routine. You'll get more in-depth information in the next chapter, but these will hold you over for now:

- **Set realistic expectations.** Understand that you can't do everything perfectly. Be kind to yourself and set realistic expectations for what you can accomplish each day.

- **Accept help.** Don't hesitate to accept help from family and friends. Whether it's watching the baby for a few hours or assisting with household chores, accepting help can give you time to recharge.

- **Delegate household tasks.** Share household responsibilities with your partner or consider hiring help if possible. This can free up time for self-care activities and prevent you from doing too much and feeling burned out.

- **Rest when you can.** Sleep deprivation is common for new parents. Nap when the baby naps, and try to go to bed early whenever possible to get enough rest.

- **Create short breaks.** Find short breaks throughout the day to do something you enjoy. Even 10 or 15 minutes of alone time to read, meditate, or take a walk can be rejuvenating.

- **Communicate with your partner.** Discuss with your partner the importance of self-care for both of you. Encourage and support each other in taking time for yourselves.

- **Stay hydrated and eat well.** Nourish your body with healthy meals and stay hydrated. Proper nutrition can make a significant difference in your energy levels and overall well-being. It's easy to get caught up in caring for your baby and not making time for your own meals, but this will quickly catch up to you and make you feel weak and unprepared for how you need to best parent your baby.

- **Exercise regularly.** Incorporate short bursts of exercise into your day, even if it's just a quick walk around the block. Exercise can boost your mood and energy levels. You can do this alone as some of your break time, or walk with the baby in a stroller or carried on your chest.

- **Connect with other parents.** Join parenting groups or online communities to connect with other new parents. Sharing experiences and advice can be uplifting. You'll find new friends who are in a similar stage of life to you and your partner, which can help you better understand parenthood and how it will change over time. You'll also have built-in friends for your baby, which can make trips to the zoo or park even more fun!

- **Practice mindfulness.** Take a few moments each day to practice mindfulness or deep breathing. It can help reduce stress and increase mental clarity. I especially recommend the 4–7–8 breathing practice when parents start to feel overwhelmed, stressed, or out of control. You inhale while counting to four, hold the breath as you count to seven, then exhale while counting to eight. It immediately calms and centers you so you can feel rejuvenated and prepared to tackle the situation that stressed you out.

- **Schedule "me time."** Set aside specific time for yourself in your daily or weekly schedule. Treat this time as sacred and nonnegotiable. This should be in addition to the time you spend with your partner as a couple because you need time alone to get back in touch with yourself in addition to staying close to your partner romantically.

- **Limit screen time.** While it's tempting to scroll through your phone during downtime, like when you're rocking the baby to sleep, excessive screen time can add to stress. You might experience a fear of missing out (FOMO) if you see posts of your friends out partying while you're sitting in a dark nursery with a baby who won't calm down. Set boundaries for screen usage and opt for more relaxing activities instead.

- **Indulge in hobbies.** Reconnect with hobbies or activities you enjoy. Whether it's painting, gardening, or playing an instrument, engaging in your passions can be therapeutic. You can do these hobbies when you have time for yourself, away from the baby, or have the baby in the same room with you. Though they're too young to understand what's going on now, as they get older they'll love hearing you play your instrument or watching you create art, and they'll appreciate that you shared your passion with them.

- **Practice self-compassion.** Parenthood is a learning curve, and it's okay to make mistakes. Be gentle with yourself and practice self-compassion. No one is perfect, so don't make yourself feel like a failure because you made a mistake or don't seem to naturally be taking to parenthood. You'll learn and adjust over time.

- **Prioritize mental health.** If you feel overwhelmed or anxious, don't hesitate to seek professional help. Talking to a therapist or counselor can provide valuable support. Just as we need to work to destigmatize postpartum mental issues, we also need to empower parents to talk to professionals when they feel like they can't cope with their daily life. Not everyone naturally takes to parenthood, and that's not a reason to feel ashamed or think you need to run away. Professionals can listen and help you feel more secure in your new role (Fletcher & Craft, 2022).

Sharing Responsibilities

Sharing responsibilities is a fundamental aspect of successful parenting for new parents. It involves collaborating with your partner to divide tasks and duties related to childcare and household management. By working as a team, you can create a supportive and balanced environment for both your child and yourselves.

My biggest recommendation to new parents is to treat newborn care like shift work. You might want to be there for every second of your baby's life, but trying to make time for that is exhausting. It's much better to take shifts with your partner—and anyone else you trust who is willing to help—to ensure you have downtime when you're not caring for the baby. Parenting can be demanding, and there may be times when you both feel overwhelmed. My method is to implement a "tag team" approach, where you take turns caring for the child, especially during challenging moments or when one parent needs a break (Klass & Damour, 2019).

For example, you may wake up with the baby on Monday and Tuesday nights, while your partner takes Wednesday and Thursday and you split the remaining days on a rotating schedule. That means each of you gets three or four full nights of sleep a week. One partner can sleep in a room away from the baby, without a baby monitor, to ensure they get quality rest. The other can sleep in the room with the baby and keep the baby monitor with them. Another example of shift work is to divide the hours. Maybe your partner handles diapers and feedings from 6 p.m. to midnight, and you handle things from midnight to 6 a.m. You can try both options to see what works for your lifestyle and schedule, or switch back and forth between methods depending on your baby's development.

Regardless of how you choose to handle overnights, effective sharing of responsibilities starts with open and honest communication. Sit down with your partner and discuss each other's expectations, strengths, and preferences in childcare and household tasks. This dialogue will help you understand each other's needs and find the best ways to distribute responsibilities. Each parent may have unique strengths and skills when it comes to parenting. Utilize these strengths to your advantage and divide responsibilities accordingly. For example, if one parent is better at organizing schedules, they could take charge of planning activities and appointments.

Parenthood involves a wide range of tasks, from feeding and changing diapers to soothing a fussy baby and managing household chores. Acknowledge and appreciate each other's contributions, no matter how small they may seem. Feeling valued and recognized enhances teamwork and motivates both parents to stay involved.

Strive for an equal partnership in parenting. This means that both parents actively participate in childcare and household duties, rather than relying heavily on one parent to take the lead. An equal partnership fosters a sense of fairness and equity in your relationship. Involve both parents in making important decisions related to your child's upbringing, education, and health. Decisions should be discussed together, considering each other's perspectives and finding common ground (Fletcher & Craft, 2022).

Both parents should have ample opportunities for bonding with the child. Participate in activities that allow you to connect individually with your little one, strengthening the parent–child relationship. But remember that you both have individual needs and interests outside of parenting. Support each other's personal time, hobbies, and self-care routines to ensure a healthy balance in your lives.

Celebrate the successes and achievements of both parents. Whether it's a small parenting win or a personal accomplishment, supporting and cheering each other on strengthens your bond as a couple. Regularly reflect on your roles as parents and assess how well you are sharing responsibilities. Be open to feedback and continuously strive for personal and parental growth.

Though you may feel tempted to dedicate as much time as possible to your child, make sure to prioritize quality time as a couple. You can nurture your relationship by spending time together without the constant focus on parenting duties. Do fun things together, ask about each other's days and hobbies, and stay connected as you did before having a child together (Karp, n.d.).

Remember that sharing responsibilities is not about being perfect or dividing tasks equally all the time. It's about working together, supporting each other, and creating a harmonious environment where both parents can thrive as they navigate the beautiful journey of parenthood.

In Our Session

If we were having a one-on-one session about becoming new parents, I would ask you questions about your adjustment during this time and how you and your partner are communicating:

- How has your communication with your partner changed since becoming parents? How do you navigate differences and make decisions together?

- How have you and your partner been supporting each other during the postpartum period? Are there ways you'd like to improve this support?

- What are some of the ways you and your partner communicate about the baby's needs and your own needs?

- How have your long-term goals and values as a couple shifted or evolved now that you're parents?

- Have you and your partner discussed your vision for the future and how you'd like to maintain a strong and healthy relationship as your family grows?

- Have you noticed any differences in how you and your partner handle disagreements or conflicts since becoming parents?

- How do you navigate conflicts to ensure they don't negatively impact your relationship or the atmosphere at home?

Chapter 5:

Becoming a New Dad

Phillip was a client who had always wanted children. He was an only child and loved the idea of a house filled with kids, toys, and noise. When Maureen told him she was pregnant, he was thrilled! He actually reached out to me during Maureen's second trimester because he wanted to get a jump start on fatherhood. I worked with them to prepare the nursery, babyproof the house, and have realistic expectations of parenthood. As an only child, Phillip had never really been around babies or experienced the sibling dynamic, so he had rose-colored glasses on during the whole pregnancy. Once his son was born, Phillip realized that babies involved a lot more care than he expected. He loved his child, but putting in so much effort made him realize that a house full of kids might be too much to handle. He wanted to be able to give each child as much attention as they needed, so we really had to work on self-care when he brought his newborn home to ensure he wouldn't burn out by giving his all to his son. It took some trial and error, but Phillip realized he could still be the best dad his son needed while making time for himself. Phillip and Maureen later had two more children, spaced out so they could fully enjoy that fleeting baby developmental period without burning out or needing to focus on another infant at the same time.

Eric grew up with an older brother and sister, both of whom had children when Eric was a teenager. He was a doting uncle, but loved being able to give the kids back to their parents when he was tired. When he married Chelsea, he knew he wanted to have a child with her, but was unsure about what type of parent he would be. He valued quiet and alone time, but didn't want to seem selfish by prioritizing that when there was a newborn in the house. Eric and Chelsea came to me during the third trimester of her pregnancy. I told them my suggestion of night shifts to prioritize sleep, and they wanted to bring that aspect of tag-teaming tasks to the rest of their parenthood journey. Chelsea didn't mind Eric having time for himself, as long as she got it too. They worked out what tasks they would take on, what they would tag-team, and how they could also spend time together as a couple. I checked in on the couple when their baby hit the two-month mark and they were running like a well-oiled machine! They both seemed well-rested and confident with who they were. Eric had worried about losing himself as he became a parent, and was astonished that he still felt like his old self.

Becoming a new dad is a life-changing and transformative experience filled with a range of emotions, challenges, and joys. It marks the beginning of a new chapter in your life, as you take on the role of a caregiver, protector, and mentor for your child. Your life starts to change as soon as you find out that your partner is pregnant. As you await the arrival of your child, you may feel a mix of excitement and anticipation. The prospect of holding your baby and embarking on this parenting journey can be both thrilling and nerve-wracking.

The arrival of a newborn can trigger a whirlwind of emotions. You might experience feelings of joy, love, anxiety, and even moments of self-doubt. Remember that these emotions are entirely normal and part of the process. The early days and weeks offer a precious opportunity to bond with your baby. Holding, cuddling, and engaging in skin-to-skin contact can strengthen the emotional connection between you and your child. As a dad, you play a crucial role in shaping your child's development. Model positive behavior, values, and communication to become a strong role model for your child as they grow, develop, and learn (N. Taylor, 2022).

New moms go through various physical and emotional changes after childbirth, as you learned in the first two chapters. Providing support and understanding, and actively participating in the care of both the baby and your partner, can be immensely valuable during this time. But remember that parenthood comes with a learning curve. From changing diapers to soothing a crying baby, you'll gradually gain confidence and become more comfortable with the routines and responsibilities of caring for your child. Parenting requires patience and adaptability. Babies have their own schedules and needs, so being flexible and patient as you adjust to your child's routine is essential.

Witnessing your baby's milestones, such as their first smile or first steps, can be incredibly rewarding. Cherish these moments and celebrate your child's achievements. Parenthood is a journey of growth, not just for your child but also for you as a dad. Embrace the challenges and joys, and savor the incredible bond that forms between you and your child.

The arrival of a baby often disrupts established routines. As a new dad, you'll need to adapt to a different sleep schedule, prioritize baby care, and balance other aspects of your life. Being a nurturing and present father involves active engagement with your child. Spend quality time playing, reading, and talking to your baby. Your involvement in their early development has a profound impact.

You also need to stay involved with your partner, especially during these early months of adjustment. Effective communication with your partner is essential as you navigate parenthood together, as you learned in the last chapter. Share your feelings, concerns, and decisions openly to build a strong parenting partnership.

Above all, remember that there's no one right way to be a dad. Each father–child relationship is unique, and your love, care, and presence in your child's life will shape them in profound ways. Embrace the joys of fatherhood and cherish every moment with your little one (Coleman, 2022).

Making the Leap From Partner to Parent

Making the leap from being a partner to becoming a parent is a transformative and profound journey. It involves a shift in roles, responsibilities, and priorities as you welcome a new life into your family. The decision to become parents is a joint commitment. Embrace this new chapter together as partners, supporting and encouraging each other every step of the way. Open and honest communication is essential during this transition. Discuss your expectations, parenting styles, and how you envision raising your child. Make plans and decisions together to create a united front in parenting.

As you step into parenthood, each of you will have different roles and responsibilities. Recognize and appreciate each other's contributions as you navigate this new terrain. Becoming parents may lead to shifts in your priorities. Your focus will now be on the well-being and needs of your child. Embrace these changes as you build a family-centered life. Parenthood comes with challenges and moments of exhaustion. Support each other emotionally and physically, allowing for breaks and self-care when needed (Coleman, 2022).

As partners, you may have different parenting approaches. It's essential to respect each other's perspectives and find common ground in making decisions for your child's upbringing. Amid the demands of parenthood, make time to be present and engaged as partners. Nurture your relationship to keep the connection strong. Embrace the learning curve of parenthood and grow together as parents. Parenthood is a journey of continuous growth and development. Both partners bring unique strengths and experiences to parenting. Learn from each other's strengths, and collaborate to create a well-rounded approach to raising your child.

Parenting can be demanding, and the responsibilities can be overwhelming at times. Share the load of childcare and household tasks to prevent burnout. Balancing your roles as parents and partners requires intention and effort. Strive to create a balance that allows you to fulfill your responsibilities as parents while nurturing your relationship as a couple. Don't hesitate to seek support from family, friends, or professional resources. Accepting help when needed can make the journey smoother. Parenthood is filled with beautiful moments and challenging ones. Embrace the entire journey, acknowledging that growth and love can emerge from both joyful and difficult experiences (N. Taylor, 2022).

Approach parenting as a team, with each partner contributing their strengths to create a supportive and loving environment for your child. Parenting is a learning process, and no one gets it perfectly right all the time. Be kind to yourselves as you navigate this new phase, and remember that you are doing your best for your child.

Making the leap from being partners to becoming parents is a significant milestone in your relationship. Embrace the joys, challenges, and growth that come with parenthood. By supporting each other, communicating openly, and cherishing your bond, you'll lay the foundation for a strong and loving family.

Parenting Fears

Parenting fears are common and natural emotions experienced by many parents. The responsibility of caring for a child and guiding their development can evoke various concerns and worries. While every parent's fears may differ based on individual circumstances and experiences, there are many common parenting fears.

Parents often fear for their child's health and safety. Worries about accidents, illnesses, and injuries can be overwhelming, especially during a child's early years when they are more vulnerable. Parents of children with health issues or disabilities may feel anxious about how to provide the best care and support for their child.

Parents may fear the impact of external influences on their child as they get older, including peer pressure and social acceptance. They want their child to be happy and accepted but worry about negative influences. As children grow, parents may worry about whether their child will perform well academically or meet societal expectations in education (Coleman, 2022).

Concerns about the future, including the challenges their child might face in terms of the status of the planet and society, can weigh heavily on parents' minds. With increasing digital exposure, parents may fear the impact of media and technology on their child's development.

New parents may fear whether they have the knowledge and skills to be good parents. Doubts about making the right decisions and providing the best care for their child can be daunting. Parents may worry about not being "good enough" or meeting societal expectations of parenting. This feeling of inadequacy can be accompanied by guilt, which arises from not being able to do everything perfectly. Parents may fear losing patience with their child during difficult moments and not being able to handle stress effectively. Fear of judgment and criticism from others about their parenting choices and methods can be a source of anxiety for some parents (Slack, 2021).

Parents often fear the challenge of balancing their work commitments with spending quality time with their child. They worry about missing out on important milestones or not being present enough.

Worries about providing for their child's needs, including education and future expenses, can be a significant stressor for parents. If you plan on having more children, or if this isn't your first baby, you may worry about fostering positive sibling relationships and maintaining a harmonious family dynamic (N. Taylor, 2022).

For new dads, the journey into parenthood can bring about a range of fears and uncertainties. While these fears may vary from one individual to another, many new dads experience common concerns as they navigate their way into fatherhood.

Some new dads fear that they might not immediately bond with their newborn or know how to connect emotionally. They may feel anxious about establishing a strong father–child bond. People focus a lot on how mothers bond with babies, and dads may feel overlooked during the newborn stage. They may think they need to stay more hands-off to allow the mother to completely bond with the baby, especially if she's breastfeeding.

New dads often worry about their lack of parenting experience and may fear not knowing how to handle different aspects of caring for a baby, such as feeding, diaper changing, or soothing. Society encourages the perception that mothers naturally know how to care for babies, so that automatically shifts the father into the "helpless" category. In reality, parenting doesn't actually come naturally, so everyone needs to learn how to feed, diaper, and soothe the baby. Dads shouldn't step back because they think the mother just naturally knows how to handle these things—they need to get active and help out, learning right along with the new mom (Coleman, 2022).

Finding a balance between work commitments and spending quality time with the baby and partner can be a significant concern for new dads. They may fear missing out on important moments and being absent during crucial stages of their child's development. There's a stereotype that dads need to go back to work immediately, leaving all the childcare and bonding to the new mom. Moms are often the ones called if the baby gets sick at daycare. They're the ones expected to come to daycare and school events because society stereotypically writes off dads as "too busy." However, this is changing, with many companies offering paternity or parental leave. Fathers are now empowered and encouraged to take time off to welcome their new baby home. I always recommend that clients who have this option take it, or use some of their vacation time if their company doesn't offer parental leave. However, many clients express that the financial responsibility of raising a child can be a major source of anxiety for new dads. They may fear whether they can provide enough for their growing family. With that in mind, they may not feel right taking time off work. I always suggest taking time, though, because you only get one chance to bond with your newborn. You can live on a budget for a few months to make it worth taking time off if you don't have paid leave, and use this time to bond with your baby and start your new family off on the right foot.

New dads may worry about adequately supporting their partner during the postpartum period. They may feel unsure about how to provide the emotional and practical support needed during this time, especially if they're still working while their partner is home on maternity leave or being a stay-at-home mother. That's where the first three chapters of this book really help you understand what your partner is going through after giving birth. While you'll never have the chance to feel what she's going through, you'll at least know what physical, mental, and emotional obstacles she may face. Understanding things from that point of view can give you an idea of what type of help she might need to rest and heal completely (Slack, 2021).

The arrival of a baby can bring changes in the dynamics of the relationship between new parents. Dads may fear how the new responsibilities will affect their relationship with their partner. Many of my clients have this fear in conjunction with the idea of supporting their partner. They worry that not understanding what their partner went through means they're not going to provide adequate support, and therefore make it more likely that their relationship will fail due to their actions—or, rather, inactions. I tell clients it's always better to err on the side of offering too much help. I think most new mothers would prefer their partner to ask to do everything for them instead of hoping he'll know what they need or having to speak up for themselves.

However, you should also feel empowered to ask for help if you need it. Your partner can still help out around the house as long as the tasks are safe for her based on the type of childbirth she experienced. You can work together or decide to hire help for certain home aspects. Hiring help is also a good way for new dads to better accept how their life will look as a parent. They may have concerns about personal sacrifices they'll have to make as a father, so temporarily outsourcing some common chores, like landscaping, mowing, and running errands, can give the new dad more time for himself and to bond with his family.

One of the biggest concerns that almost every new dad client has had is regarding emotions. Just like paternity leave being a relatively new development in our culture, men showing emotions is also rare and not always encouraged. Some new dads may fear expressing their emotions openly, feeling societal pressure to be strong or not show vulnerability. They think they need to present a solid, masculine exterior to be a respectable father. However, fathers often feel emotional with their children, especially when you witness your baby coming into this world. I tell male clients that it's never wrong to cry at that moment because it truly feels like a miracle, and you realize how much of an impact this little baby has on your life, your self, and everything around you. Becoming a father truly changes people, so it's a great opportunity to start sharing your emotions with your baby and partner, and others if you feel comfortable (Coleman, 2022).

When you're more open with your emotions, you'll find that you feel more connected to others. Trying to hide your emotions will make you feel isolated and it feels tough to relate to others. You need support during the early stages of parenthood to keep you on the right path, help you with practical advice, and feel connected with people around you. It's too easy to get consumed by your new family and close yourself off to others, so external support will prevent this (Slack, 2021).

It's essential for new dads to recognize that it's normal to have fears and concerns about parenting. Seeking support from their partner, family, and friends, as well as joining parenting groups or seeking professional guidance, can be beneficial in navigating these uncertainties. With time, patience, and an open heart, new dads can develop the confidence and skills to be loving and effective fathers to their children.

The Importance of Self-Care

You knew this section was coming. I kept mentioning it because my clients often think they need to work themselves to the bone for their new baby. They think if they give their all, things will work out fine. However, they don't realize that putting all of yourself into your baby leaves nothing else for you or your partner. I always go back to the concept of helping others on a plane. You have to put your own oxygen mask on first, otherwise you won't be around to help anyone else. While many things in parenting require you to put the baby first, that doesn't mean you forget yourself. Sure, you can feed the baby before you sit down for a meal, but you don't skip that meal to then go read a story to your baby. You'll feel tired and lack the energy needed to engage with your baby, so you need to eat while they play independently, and then you can read to them.

Amid all the demands of caring for a newborn, you can't forget to prioritize self-care. Taking care of your physical and mental well-being will help you be a more patient and present father. This may include asking for help from family or friends. Parenthood can be overwhelming, and having a support system can make a significant difference. You won't feel alone as you learn how to care for a newborn. You can get advice from the people you trust to help you out, or you might want to use that time as a break. Leave the house to clear your head. Go for a walk or drive and spend some time alone with your thoughts (N. Taylor, 2022).

The importance of self-care for new parents cannot be overstated. While the demands of caring for a newborn may seem all-consuming, taking care of yourself is crucial for your well-being and your ability to be the best parent you can be. Self-care helps you maintain your physical health. Adequate rest, proper nutrition, and regular exercise are essential to keep your energy levels up and support your body as you care for your child (Slack, 2021).

The early days of parenthood can be emotionally challenging. Self-care practices like mindfulness, meditation, or seeking professional support can help reduce stress, anxiety, and feelings of overwhelm. When you take time for self-care, you recharge emotionally and mentally. This can lead to increased patience and a greater ability to handle the challenges that come with parenting. Parenting can be exhausting, especially in the early stages. Regular self-care helps prevent burnout and allows you to approach parenting with a refreshed and positive mindset (Coleman, 2022).

By prioritizing self-care, you model healthy habits for your child. They learn that it's essential to take care of yourself to maintain overall well-being. They'll see this as they get older, but they'll also feel it even as babies and toddlers. When you're taking care of yourself, you are more present and engaged when spending time with your child. This quality time strengthens your bond and promotes a positive parent–child relationship. Taking time for self-care allows your child to develop a sense of independence and self-soothing skills, as they learn to spend some time without constant attention.

When you're well-rested and emotionally balanced, you can approach challenges with clearer thinking and better problem-solving skills. Engaging in self-care activities that bring you joy and fulfillment can provide a sense of rejuvenation and renewal, making you better equipped to face daily responsibilities. Self-care builds emotional resilience, helping you cope better during tough times and bounce back from difficult situations. Parental burnout is a real phenomenon that can lead to feelings of detachment and emotional exhaustion. Self-care acts as a preventative measure against burnout.

Engaging in self-care activities that make you feel good about yourself can boost your self-esteem and overall sense of well-being. Parenthood is a significant life change, but it doesn't mean you should lose your individual identity. Self-care helps you maintain a sense of self amid the responsibilities of parenting. Just as you nurture your child, it's essential to nurture yourself. Self-care is an act of self-love and self-compassion.

Remember that self-care doesn't have to be elaborate or time-consuming. Even small moments of self-care, like taking a short walk, reading a book, or enjoying a quiet cup of tea, can have a positive impact on your well-being. Prioritizing self-care as a new parent is an investment in your health, happiness, and ability to be the loving and attentive parent your child needs. This list is just an idea of self-care options you might choose as a new parent, but feel free to come up with your own ideas based on what priorities and hobbies you have in your life (Slack, 2021):

- **Take short breaks.** Find short moments throughout the day to take breaks. Even a few minutes of quiet time to breathe deeply or step outside can help you recharge.

- **Get enough sleep.** As a new parent, sleep might be limited, but prioritize rest whenever possible. Take turns with your partner for night feedings and naps during the day to catch up on sleep.

- **Exercise regularly.** Engage in physical activities that you enjoy, such as jogging, cycling, or playing sports. Exercise not only improves physical health but also reduces stress and boosts mood.

- **Connect with other dads.** Join a dads' support group or connect with other fathers. Sharing experiences and advice with fellow dads can be uplifting and validating.

- **Practice mindfulness.** Take a few minutes each day to practice mindfulness or meditation. It can help reduce stress and increase your ability to be present in the moment.

- **Engage in a hobby.** Set aside time for a hobby or activity you enjoy. Whether it's reading, drawing, playing a musical instrument, playing sports, or woodworking, doing something you love can be rejuvenating.

- **Support your partner's self-care.** Encourage and support your partner in her self-care routine as well. Working together to prioritize self-care can benefit both of you.

- **Stay connected with friends.** Maintain social connections with friends and engage in activities outside of parenthood. Socializing can be refreshing and energizing.

- **Write in a journal.** Consider keeping a journal to jot down your thoughts and feelings. Writing can be a therapeutic way to process emotions and reflect on your parenting journey.

- **Learn something new.** Challenge yourself to learn something new, whether it's a new recipe, a DIY project, or a skill you've always wanted to master.

- **Go for walks with your baby.** Taking a walk with your baby in a stroller or carrier not only provides fresh air for both of you but also offers an opportunity for bonding.

- **Laugh and have fun.** Don't forget to have fun and find moments to laugh with your child. Playfulness can be therapeutic and strengthen your bond.

In Our Session

If we were having a one-on-one session about becoming a new dad, I'd ask how you were bonding with the baby while caring for yourself:

- How do you feel your bond with the baby is developing? Are there specific moments or activities that have helped strengthen this bond?

- Do you feel comfortable and confident in your interactions with the baby? Are there areas where you'd like to improve your caregiving skills?

- What strategies have you been using to take care of yourself during this period of adjustment? How do you ensure you're getting enough rest and maintaining your well-being?

- Have you found it challenging to establish boundaries between your new role as a father and your personal interests and responsibilities? How do you manage this balance?

- What activities or practices help you relax and manage stress? How frequently are you engaging in these activities?

- How do you handle situations where you feel overwhelmed or frustrated? Are there any coping strategies you'd like to explore further?

Chapter 6:

Relationship Changes

Having children is a major life change, and you're going to go through a lot of changes and growth in the process. So will your relationship—for better or for worse.

Dale and Christina had been married for five years before they felt ready to have a baby. They loved each other and were excited to start a family, so they hired me early on in the pregnancy. We went over all the issues first-time parents may face so they would have an idea of the roller coaster they could face—or not! Some people naturally take to parenthood and work together like a well-oiled machine. And that was Dale and Christina, though I can't say it came naturally. They definitely put in the work and prepared themselves for every possible outcome. If parenthood was an exam, they would have out-studied anyone else taking the test! But this level of preparedness was what made them feel most comfortable, so it was the right choice for them. When their son was born, they already had a shift schedule to ensure everyone would get the sleep needed. They had prepared the nursery, stockpiled supplies, and had meals stored in the freezer. They staggered family and friend visits to allow everyone to meet the baby at times that didn't wear out the new parents—and possibly even gave them time to shower or nap! Everything worked smoothly and Christina healed during the fourth trimester, thanks to help from Dave and their extensive support system.

I first met Mark and Bailey when their daughter was a month old. They had prepared the nursery and, after almost a decade together, felt like they were ready for anything. However, they were so used to being a fun couple—traveling extensively, dining out, and perfecting custom cocktails—that staying home and being parents was a rude awakening. Though they knew each other completely and loved each other, they were used to being a family of two. Having a newborn shifted their priorities in a way they hadn't expected. Everyone knows that becoming a parent means you have to put the baby first, but for this couple, it meant that they totally lost themselves. They each functioned independently. While they fed, bathed, cleaned, and bonded with the baby, they didn't make time to reconnect as a couple. They started to resent each other because they weren't communicating or functioning as a team. After a month, they felt like they were failing as parents and losing themselves. I talked to them about what they missed most from being a couple. Surprisingly, it wasn't dining out at the hottest restaurants in town or flying around the globe whenever they had time off. They missed taking time to sit with each other and talk. They wanted to laugh and feel connected instead of feeling like they only existed to care for their daughter. We prioritized date nights and put an hour on their calendar each night after the baby went to bed. They could talk, laugh, make dinner, craft custom cocktails, or do whatever they wanted in that hour—but they had to do it as a couple. Knowing that they were able to put aside their parental personas for a few hours each week helped them understand how they could balance their relationship with their daughter. It was a bit of a learning curve, but making the leap from a couple to a family is something you can navigate and grow from.

Going From Partners to Parents—Together

Becoming new parents can bring significant changes to a relationship. While it's an exciting and fulfilling journey, it can also be challenging and demanding. The arrival of a baby often shifts the couple's priorities. The focus may shift from each other to the needs and well-being of the baby. This can lead to less time and attention being devoted to the relationship, causing some strain.

Sleep deprivation and increased responsibilities can affect communication between partners. It may become harder to find time to talk and connect on a deeper level. Misunderstandings may occur due to exhaustion and stress. New parents may experience conflicts over the division of childcare and household responsibilities. Each partner might have different expectations or ideas about how things should be done, which can lead to tension and arguments. Both partners may experience a range of emotions, including joy, love, frustration, and stress. Adjusting to the new role of being parents can be emotionally overwhelming. This can add to communication issues in ways you never experienced before bringing a baby into the home.

The physical and emotional demands of caring for a baby can impact a couple's intimacy and sex life. The lack of time, energy, and sometimes body image concerns can affect the couple's closeness. Depending on the type of childbirth your wife experiences, you may not be able to have sex for about six weeks. You can always ask your medical provider for clarification, but your wife needs time to heal without risking injury or infection. Some women experience vaginal dryness or increased sensitivity after giving birth, and may feel reluctant to have intercourse. You can talk to your partner to ensure they're comfortable with the idea of having sex again, including using lubrication to prevent discomfort. However, there are other ways to be intimate. Starting slowly is the best way to get back into the swing of a physical relationship. You'll be able to foster an emotional connection to increase intimacy before jumping into physical action. You can also make time to cuddle, hug, kiss, touch, and partake in activities that don't require penetration. The timing and experience of resuming sexual activity after childbirth vary for each individual. Some couples may feel ready to engage in sexual intimacy relatively quickly, while others may need more time. The key is to communicate openly, be patient with yourself and your partner, and prioritize your well-being and the well-being of your baby.

The added expenses related to raising a child can put a strain on the family's finances. Financial worries may lead to disagreements between partners. There are also discussions about going back to work, enrolling the baby in daycare, and trying to manage the disruptions all this causes to your schedules. The cost of daycare alone can be a big source of tension for couples, especially if that expense will wipe out one partner's paycheck. Keeping an open line of communication and not judging each other during these discussions can go a long way toward strengthening your relationship. One partner may want to stay home with the baby, at least for a few years, instead of sinking so much money into daycare. However, many people enjoy working outside of the home and feel a sense of accomplishment from their job, even if they'll be working to pay for daycare. There is no one set solution for childcare and employment, so talking with your partner can make a big difference in your financial stress and communication levels.

As parents, both partners may experience shifts in their roles and identities. This adjustment can be both fulfilling and challenging. You're a new father and your partner is a new mother. It's easy to feel overwhelmed at this new responsibility. Many people have told me that they start to see their partner in a different light, which can be good or bad! Seeing your partner care for your baby may make you feel a rush of love and attraction for them. Or you might start seeing them as a provider to the baby instead of your partner in life, and you feel a disconnect in your relationship. These roles can change often over your child's lifetime, so being flexible and openly communicating with your partner can make the process much easier.

While these changes can be difficult, they are also a natural part of the transition to parenthood. It's essential for new parents to communicate openly and honestly about their feelings, needs, and concerns. These tips will help you navigate these changes together:

- Make time for regular communication, even if it's just a few minutes each day to check in and share your thoughts and feelings. Talk openly with your partner about your feelings, fears, and expectations regarding parenthood. Be honest about any concerns you may have and listen to your partner's thoughts as well.

- Work together to find a fair and balanced way to divide childcare and household responsibilities. Consider each other's strengths and preferences. Work together as a team instead of putting the bulk of responsibilities on one person. Be open to re-evaluating and adjusting the division as needed.

- Don't hesitate to ask for help from family or friends when needed. Building a support system is crucial. You also need to be supportive of each other and offer help when needed. Remember that you're both learning and adapting to this new experience.

- Find ways to nurture your physical and emotional connection. Even small gestures of affection and appreciation can go a long way. Although the demands of parenting can be overwhelming, it's crucial to set aside time for just the two of you. Plan date nights or find moments for simple acts of connection, like having a cup of tea together after the baby has gone to sleep.

- Be open to adapting and adjusting your expectations. Parenthood is a learning process and flexibility is essential. Recognize and appreciate the efforts your partner puts into parenting. Whether it's changing diapers, soothing the baby, or preparing meals, acknowledging each other's contributions helps create a positive atmosphere in the relationship.

- Remember to take care of your own well-being. Taking care of yourself will enable you to better support your partner and your child. Taking care of yourselves individually will positively impact your ability to care for your child and each other. Prioritize self-care and encourage your partner to do the same.

- Embrace the joys of parenthood as a team. Participate in parenting activities together, such as reading bedtime stories, going on family outings, and creating new traditions. Celebrate the joys and milestones of your child together. Be there for each other during the challenging times as well. Share the emotional journey of parenthood as partners.

- If you find that the changes are causing significant distress, consider seeking support from a therapist or counselor who specializes in couples' and family dynamics.

It's normal for relationships to undergo changes during this transformative period. With understanding, patience, and support, many couples find that these changes strengthen their bond and create a deeper level of connection as they navigate the joys and challenges of parenthood together. As long as you're keeping communication open with your partner and working toward a happy, productive life, you're going to be on the right track as parents and as a couple. You can also seek professional help to iron out the kinks if there is love at the foundation.

Your Wife Is a New Mom

Your loving relationship with your wife has led both of you to embrace the beautiful journey of becoming parents. However, what many partners may not anticipate is the shift from a focus on "the two of us" to the inclusion of your newborn, which can pose challenges. Despite the excitement surrounding this momentous occasion, it's crucial to recognize that once the little one arrives, your wife's focus, time, attention, and energy will naturally be directed toward the baby rather than solely on you. Striking the right balance during this transition is essential to ensure a smooth adjustment for everyone involved, ensuring that no one feels left out in this new chapter of your lives.

The moment a woman becomes a new mom marks a profound transformation in her life. With the arrival of a baby, she embarks on an incredible journey of motherhood, where her role becomes central to the well-being of her child. As the baby's primary caregiver, she holds the responsibility of meeting their every need and nurturing them through the early stages of life. This newfound role can be both rewarding and overwhelming as she navigates the challenges and joys of motherhood. Oh, and don't forget—you're along for the ride! It can feel tough to watch her be the primary caregiver for your baby, but first, let's look at things from her point of view.

The Baby Is Dependent on Her

As a new mom, her baby becomes her priority. The little one relies on her for everything, from nourishment and comfort to safety and love. This level of dependency can create an intense bond between mother and child, but it also means that her attention and time may be almost entirely consumed by the baby's needs. Balancing the demands of caring for an infant with other aspects of her life can be a delicate task, one that requires understanding and support from you as her partner.

If your wife breastfeeds the baby, you may feel like you can't participate in that part of their lives. However, open communication is key. Your wife may prefer to be alone with the baby while they nurse so the baby isn't distracted by your presence. It's also a great bonding opportunity for the two of them. Some women don't mind having their partner nearby, though, because they have a chance to talk. Some women may also want to pump milk so you can bottle-feed the baby—though this can be difficult and frustrating for some mothers, so don't push the issue if your wife can't pump enough milk. If your baby still seems hungry, you could talk about adding formula to supplement the breast milk, and take on the role of feeding the baby formula so your wife gets a break from being the baby's sole provider of food.

Though your wife may be the baby's primary caretaker, it doesn't have to be that way—especially during the fourth trimester, when she needs to rest and heal. Many new dads step back because they think their wife wants to be the sole provider, or they assume she just naturally knows how to feed, change, and bathe the baby. But you're both learning together, so help out whenever you can. Talk with your wife about what tasks you can do to take the stress off of her while she recovers. Make sure she knows the baby isn't dependent only on her—that you're there to care for both of them in any way you can.

As a dad, supporting a new mom who feels overwhelmed by the baby's dependence on her is crucial in creating a positive and nurturing environment for both the mother and the child. Acknowledge and validate your wife's feelings of being overwhelmed and reassure her that it's normal to feel this way. Let her know that you understand the challenges she is facing and that you are there to support her. Educate yourself about baby care, so you feel confident and capable in assisting with the baby's needs. Understanding the baby's routines and preferences can make it easier for you to step in and support your wife. Offer to help with the baby's care, such as diaper changes, feeding, and soothing. Sharing the responsibilities of caring for the baby can provide her with much-needed breaks and help her feel less overwhelmed. It also gives you both the chance to bond with the baby while still getting rest. Encourage bonding time between her and the baby but create opportunities for you to bond with the baby as well. Skin-to-skin contact, holding the baby, and participating in activities like bath time can help foster your relationship with the baby.

If your wife feels like the primary caregiver, she may put the baby's needs above her own. Remind her to take breaks and prioritize self-care. Encourage her to rest, eat well, and engage in activities that bring her joy. Taking care of herself will help her recharge and be better equipped to care for the baby. Take on extra household chores to ease her workload. Keeping the house tidy and organized can reduce her stress and allow her to focus more on the baby.

In addition to providing assistance with the baby's needs, make yourself available when your wife needs you. Be there to listen and provide emotional support. Let her know that she can talk to you about her feelings, fears, and frustrations without judgment. Discuss your roles and responsibilities as parents openly and find a balance that works for both of you. Regularly check in with each other to ensure you are both feeling supported and heard. Acknowledge and celebrate each other's efforts and successes as parents. Recognize the challenges you both overcome and the milestones achieved by the baby.

If necessary, consider seeking the support of family, friends, or professional services, such as postpartum doulas or support groups. Having an additional support system can be beneficial for both of you. The transition to parenthood is a learning process for both of you, and it's okay to make mistakes and learn together. Your support, understanding, and willingness to be actively involved will make a significant difference in helping the new mom feel less overwhelmed and more confident in her role as a mother. Together, you can create a loving and nurturing environment for your growing family.

She May Feel Guilty

Ironically, as much as she devotes herself to caring for the baby, a new mom may experience feelings of guilt and inadequacy. Amid the sleepless nights, diaper changes, and constant feedings, she might wonder if she is doing enough or if she should be doing more. This guilt can stem from the sense of responsibility she feels for her child's well-being and her own desire to be the best mother possible. Society makes it seem like the only good mothers are those who completely give themselves up to their baby. But if your wife does that, she may feel like she's only around to provide for the baby, and she'll stop feeling like herself. During the fourth trimester, this is a delicate balance. You want her to feel like a good mother without feeling overwhelmed, lost, and depressed.

Dads play a crucial role in supporting new moms and helping them feel less guilty about their motherhood journey. Regularly express your gratitude and appreciation for all the hard work and care she puts into being a mother. Let her know that you see and value her efforts. Remind her that her role as a mother is irreplaceable and that she plays a vital role in your child's life. Emphasize how much your child loves and needs her. Demonstrate your trust in her abilities as a mother. Allow her to make decisions about parenting and support her choices.

Be actively involved in caring for the baby and the household. Show that you are a committed and engaged partner in parenthood, and share the responsibilities equally. Let her know that she can ask you for any type of help and you'll step up. Also stay available for her to talk to you when she needs to vent or feel reassured that she's doing a great job adjusting to parenthood. Create an environment where she feels comfortable expressing her feelings and concerns without judgment. Listen actively and be supportive when she shares her thoughts. When she expresses doubts or guilt, reassure her that all parents face challenges and that it's normal to feel uncertain at times. Remind her that you are there to navigate this journey together.

Compliment her parenting skills and the bond she shares with the baby. Point out the positive moments you observe between her and your child. Celebrate the baby's milestones together as a team. Acknowledge the growth and development of your child and recognize how her care and love have contributed to these achievements. Plan special moments for the three of you to bond as a family. Whether it's going for a walk, reading a story together, or cuddling, these shared experiences can strengthen your family bond.

Remember that adjusting to motherhood is a significant life change, and it takes time to adapt. Be patient with her as she navigates this new role. Encourage her to take time for herself and engage in activities she enjoys. Offer to care for the baby while she takes a break or spends time doing something that rejuvenates her.

Building confidence as a new mom is an ongoing process. Your consistent support, understanding, and encouragement will go a long way in helping her feel less guilty and more assured in her role as a loving and capable mother. Together, you can create a nurturing and loving environment for your child to thrive.

It's Not Just the Two of Us

Adjusting to a new baby, and transitioning from being part of a couple to becoming parents, is a significant life change for new parents. New mothers are often consumed with caring for the newborn while dads might feel out of place and unsure of how and when to step in and provide care for their wife and the baby. It helps to actively participate in caring for the baby from the beginning. Get involved in diaper changes, feeding, soothing, and playtime. Being present and engaged in the baby's daily routines will help you bond with your child and feel more confident as a dad. You'll help your wife and show her that you're prepared to take on any role necessary. This will give her more time to rest, relax, and heal, which will ensure she continues feeling your love even as she adjusts to being a mother.

Open communication with your partner is essential during this time of adjustment. Share your thoughts, feelings, and concerns with each other. Discuss your roles and responsibilities as parents and find ways to support each other. Instead of letting issues fester, talk about them. Even if you feel like you don't know how to help care for the baby, talk to your wife about it so she knows you'd like to be more involved. Talking with her will help you see what she struggles with and how you can make things easier on her, which will help her feel loved and prioritize your relationship while you both care for the baby.

To ensure you can help your wife and baby the most, take the time to learn about baby care, infant development, and parenting techniques. Reading books, attending parenting classes, or seeking advice from experienced parents can help you feel more prepared and competent. If you don't think you know how to change a diaper correctly, ask your wife for tips or watch what she does so you can learn from her. Better yet, if you don't know the answer to an issue, look it up and try to solve it yourself instead of putting the responsibility on your wife to teach you.

If possible, take advantage of paternity leave or explore flexible work arrangements to spend more time with your new baby. This dedicated time together will help you establish a strong bond. During that time, you can be the primary caregiver for your baby so your wife can heal. Prioritize special bonding time with your baby. Engage in activities like baby massage, singing, reading, or playing together. These shared experiences will strengthen your connection and build trust with your child. You can also make time together as a couple. While the focus shifts to the baby, it's essential to prioritize your relationship with your partner. Find time for intimate moments, date nights, or simple conversations to nurture your connection. Above all, be flexible and adaptable as you navigate the unpredictable nature of parenting. Embracing change and being open to new experiences will help you adjust more effectively.

Acknowledge the physical and emotional challenges your partner may face during the postpartum period. Offer emotional support, assist with household tasks, and encourage her to prioritize self-care. Many men realize that childbirth is a major experience, but don't talk about it with their partner or express their admiration. Doing so will help your partner feel confident, appreciated, and loved.

Every parent's journey is unique, and it's okay to experience a mix of emotions during this transition. By actively engaging in your child's care, supporting your partner, and seeking help when needed, you will find your way to becoming a loving and nurturing father. Your love and presence in your child's life will have a profound impact on their growth and development.

How to Navigate the Transition

Parenthood is a learning process, and it's normal to encounter challenges along the way. Be patient with yourself, your partner, and your baby—this is new for all of you! Embrace flexibility and adaptability as you adjust to the new role. Parenthood can be filled with unexpected and sometimes humorous moments. Embrace the humor and find joy in the little things. Stay curious and educate yourselves about parenting, child development, and each other's needs. Continuously learning and growing as parents will benefit your child and your relationship.

Prioritize self-care for both parents. Get enough rest, eat well, and engage in activities that rejuvenate you. Taking care of yourselves will help you be better parents. Find moments to spend quality time together as a couple and as a family. It doesn't have to be elaborate; even small moments of connection can make a difference. While your baby is a priority, remember to nurture your romantic relationship. Make time for each other and show appreciation and affection.

Don't hesitate to ask for help from family, friends, or support groups. Surround yourself with a support network that can offer advice, encouragement, and assistance when needed.

Navigating becoming a new dad while prioritizing your romantic relationship requires a delicate balance between parenthood and partnership. You can feel torn between prioritizing your baby or your relationship, and it's hard to say one way is better than the other. You're a loving couple who brought a baby into the world, so you want to strengthen your love even more during this time. However, the baby needs all the help they can get, so you need to ensure their needs are met, which creates a balancing act. Taking shifts for baby care can greatly help you both feel like you have downtime, a chance to bond with the baby, and time to communicate with each other once the baby is sleeping. Try to carve out time each week to be with your partner, whether it's after the baby goes to bed or when a trusted friend or family member watches the baby for a few hours so you and your wife can enjoy a date night. It might seem like a time crunch to schedule all this, but remember that things will change as your baby gets older. By prioritizing your relationship now, you're giving yourselves a stronger foundation to rely on as your family grows and changes.

By working together as partners and parents, you can create a loving and nurturing environment for your baby and maintain a strong, supportive relationship with each other. Remember that the journey of parenthood is a shared experience, and the love and care you both provide will shape your child's life in a profound way. Every family is different and there's no one way to be a parent. You and your wife will learn how to work together to create the best life for your baby while still prioritizing each other and loving every moment of your lives together.

In Our Session

If we were having a one-on-one session about changes to your relationship, I would ask you about what you've noticed or felt in your relationship since bringing your baby home, including communication, responsibilities, and intimacy:

- How would you describe the changes you've noticed in your relationship with your partner since becoming parents?

- What aspects of your relationship have remained stable, and what aspects have shifted?

- How has communication between you and your partner evolved since the arrival of your baby?

- Have you and your partner found new ways to connect and spend quality time together? How do you maintain a strong emotional bond amid the demands of parenting?

- How have you and your partner divided responsibilities related to caregiving and household tasks? How does this division impact your relationship and sense of partnership?

- Have you experienced any challenges or conflicts related to managing shared responsibilities? How do you work through these challenges together?

- How has the physical aspect of your relationship, including intimacy, changed since becoming parents?

- What are some of the factors that contribute to maintaining intimacy in your relationship amid the demands of parenthood?

- How do you and your partner prioritize self-care and time for yourselves while also nurturing your relationship?

- Have you been able to find a balance between your roles as parents and your roles as partners?

Chapter 7:

Action Plan

I've had many clients who think that, because childbirth is natural, they don't need to plan. I can't tell you how wrong this is! Yes, a woman's body knows what to do during childbirth, but that's when everything goes well. I always recommend having a plan, and then a backup plan, while also being flexible enough to have a few other options in mind in case nothing else works out.

Ronnie and Megan always flew by the seats of their pants—literally! Ronnie was a pilot and Megan was a freelancer so they were always ready to take a trip whenever Ronnie had a flight with an extra seat for Megan. With that life experience forming the base for their relationship, they had learned to roll with the punches. They were used to traveling with one backpack each, making do with whatever accommodations they could find while they were already on the road. Because they were so flexible, they knew that whatever happened during childbirth and postpartum, they'd be able to handle it. Since Megan was a freelancer, she figured she'd just work fewer hours after the baby was born so she could stay home with the baby while still earning money for the family. Ronnie was taking a week off of work but would be piloting flights again after that point, so Megan's ability to stay home was crucial. They took their time setting up the nursery, but Megan went into labor early, before Ronnie had even constructed the crib! In the hospital, the couple found out that the baby was breech and in distress, so Megan needed a C-section. Thankfully, the labor went well and Megan and the baby only needed to stay in the hospital for three additional days—which gave Ronnie time to finish putting the crib together! However, when the new family went home, they realized Ronnie couldn't go back to work because Megan needed to heal from her C-section wound. She couldn't raise her arms over her head or lift things, so Ronnie had to do everything for her. And because she needed so much rest to heal, Megan couldn't do her freelance work. The couple scrambled to get everything together to ensure both mama and baby had the care they needed, but it was a rough few weeks. While their ability to think on their feet and be flexible made a big difference in their demeanor during that postpartum period, if they had planned ahead, they might have been better prepared for what could possibly come their way. While no one knows how labor will go and a breech baby can always surprise you, having a plan and a backup plan can go a long way toward ensuring you have your bases covered for a less-than-ideal scenario.

Naomi and Conner were a super-organized couple who met with me almost as soon as they got the positive pregnancy test! I'm joking of course, but only slightly. This couple loved having their lives planned out. They both worked long hours at high-stress jobs, so they carefully planned late-night dinners together, plus time on the weekends for dates and togetherness. They saved their vacation time to make the most of opportunities to go abroad and spend weeks in stunning destinations. They were so excited to have a baby, but the uncertainty of it all threw them for a loop. They came to me wanting to know every possible outcome. They'd ask, "What would it be like if we scheduled a C-section?" and I'd give them a few possible scenarios, like I've done at the start of each chapter of this book. But then I'd ask them, "What if the baby comes naturally before the scheduled C-section?" They'd go back to the drawing board and come up with another plan for that option. We kept meeting until they felt like they had considered every possibility. They had plans for parental leave from work and had already negotiated a low return to the office, including time working from home as the baby transitioned into daycare. I feel like a very organized person, but Naomi and Conner put me to shame! That said, as these things often happen, everything went according to plan! The baby held on until Naomi's scheduled C-section and there were no hiccups along the way. The baby's nursery was ready ahead of time and the family visits were all planned in ways that would help the new parents rest up without stress. I thought the couple would be frustrated that they'd spent so much time worrying about what never happened, but the opposite was true! They were glad they had prepared and thought about all the options so nothing would take them by surprise. Plus, Conner told me later, they didn't have to cook for months because they had so many frozen meals and scheduled meal trains! So there's certainly a benefit to planning ahead, even if you don't need to follow any of those alternate paths.

There's a reason you should create an action plan. Childbirth and the postpartum period can be overwhelming for new parents due to the physical, emotional, and lifestyle changes that come with bringing a new life into the world. The responsibilities of caring for a newborn, combined with sleep deprivation and hormonal fluctuations, can create significant challenges for new parents. To help cope with this overwhelming time, creating an action plan can be beneficial because you don't have to stop and think of what to do each time something happens. You have a planned path to follow, so you can just check the plan and continue on without having to stress yourself about finding a solution.

Before the baby arrives, educate yourselves about childbirth, postpartum recovery, and newborn care. Attend prenatal classes, read books, and consult with health-care professionals to gain a better understanding of what to expect. Reach out to family, friends, or other parents who can provide emotional support, practical advice, or a helping hand when needed. Having a strong support network can make a significant difference during this time. Arrange for someone to assist with household chores or cooking during the early postpartum period. This will allow you to focus on rest and bonding with the baby.

Set up the nursery, organize baby essentials, and ensure your home is safe and babyproofed. This preparation can help reduce stress once the baby is born. But even if you have everything set up, understand that newborns have unpredictable schedules, and it's essential to be flexible with your routines. Focus on feeding the baby on demand and allow for plenty of rest and naps for both the baby and parents.

Open communication is vital during this time. Discuss responsibilities, emotions, and any challenges you are facing. Support each other and work as a team in caring for the baby. Ensure both of you get enough rest, eat nutritious meals, and engage in light exercise if possible. Postpartum recovery can take time, so be patient with yourselves. You should make time for activities that bring you joy and relaxation. This can be anything from reading a book to taking a short walk or practicing mindfulness exercises.

If either of you experiences feelings of overwhelm, anxiety, or depression that persist for weeks, seek help from a health-care provider or mental health professional. PPD and postpartum anxiety are common and should be addressed promptly. Early detection can go a long way in ensuring everyone in your family stays mentally, emotionally, and physically healthy, so don't wait to talk to your doctor or a therapist if something seems off. And remember that this is the prime time to accept help from others, even if you're used to being independent or being the one to help everyone else. You might want help taking care of the baby for a few hours so you and your partner can sleep, get out of the house, or have some alone time. Help with meals, groceries, errands, and household chores will also greatly impact how you adapt to new parenthood, so try to add this into your action plan.

Remember, every parent's journey is unique, and it's okay to have challenging days. Being kind to yourself and recognizing that it's okay to ask for support will go a long way in navigating the overwhelming aspects of childbirth and the postpartum period, even if you already have an action plan in place. This should serve as a guideline you can use when you're unable to get your head together enough to think straight, but isn't something you need to stick to if situations change.

Clear Ideas for an Awesome Postpartum Experience

Childbirth and the postpartum period can be incredibly overwhelming for new parents. The physical and emotional changes that come with becoming parents, coupled with the demands of caring for a newborn, can lead to stress and exhaustion. To navigate this transformative phase successfully, it's essential to create a well-thought-out action plan that addresses key aspects before, during, and after birth.

Before Birth

You're probably thrilled when you find out your partner is pregnant, but then you realize there's a lot to do in just nine short months! Preparing for the arrival of your baby is an exciting and essential time. Creating a well-organized action plan can help you feel more confident and ready for the changes that come with becoming a parent.

Find a Medical Provider

In the early stages, you can research and select a health-care provider. Look into both obstetrician-gynecologists (OB/GYNs) and midwives, depending on your preference for medical treatment. Choosing between an OB/GYN and a midwife for your prenatal care and childbirth is a personal decision that depends on various factors. Each group of professionals has different approaches to pregnancy and childbirth, and your specific needs and preferences will play a significant role in making this choice. I've had many clients who experience anxiety and high blood pressure when going to doctor's offices or the hospital, so they prefer using a midwife, who has a more laid-back approach to prenatal care and childbirth. However, that doesn't diminish their experience and expertise. You can find Certified Nurse Midwives who can handle the same medical procedures as a doctor. If your partner has a high-risk pregnancy or a history of medical complications, an OB/GYN may be more appropriate. They have extensive medical training and can handle complex pregnancies and childbirth.

Consider your personal philosophy on childbirth. Midwives often focus on a more holistic, patient-centered approach, emphasizing natural childbirth and promoting a woman's autonomy during labor. OB/GYNs, on the other hand, are trained in both medical and surgical interventions and may be more inclined to recommend medical interventions if needed. If you have a preference for a natural birth with minimal medical intervention, a midwife may be a good fit. Midwives are often associated with birthing centers or home births, where they provide continuous support throughout labor. Midwives often offer a more personalized and continuous model of care. They typically spend more time with their patients and may be available for more extended periods during labor. You might also be able to retain your midwife during the postpartum period and have easier access to getting help and answers from her compared to a doctor. In some cases, you may have the option of a team approach, where both an OB/GYN and a midwife work together to provide care during pregnancy and childbirth. This can combine the benefits of both approaches. Regardless of the type of provider you choose, schedule regular prenatal checkups to monitor your baby's growth and ensure your partner and your baby's well-being.

Prioritize Health

Your partner can begin taking prenatal vitamins with folic acid as recommended by her health-care provider to support her health and the baby's development. You can ensure she eats a balanced diet, stays hydrated, and engages in moderate exercise approved by her health-care provider. You should both avoid smoking, alcohol, and illicit drugs to create a healthy home environment for your bundle of joy.

Make Financial Decisions

Check your health insurance policy to understand coverage for prenatal care, birth, and postpartum care. Explore additional policies or plans if needed. Plan your finances for baby-related expenses, including nursery setup, baby gear, medical costs, and potential parental leave.

Discuss maternity/paternity leave options with your employer and plan for time off after the baby's birth. Whether you have time off or not, you may also want to coordinate with family or friends who can assist you during the initial postpartum period with cooking, cleaning, or caring for the baby.

Educate Yourself

Attend prenatal classes that address childbirth, breastfeeding, postpartum care, and newborn care. You'll learn what can happen during childbirth and what life will actually look like once you bring home your baby. Read books and seek advice from health-care professionals to understand the birthing process and postpartum care better. Knowledge can help ease anxiety and boost confidence so you feel prepared when the baby comes. This concept of knowledge includes discussing birthing preferences with your health-care provider, outlining preferences for pain management, medical interventions, and any other specific desires for the birth experience. You can also use this time to build a support system of family and friends who can provide emotional support and practical assistance during and after childbirth. People who are parents may have good advice you can use now, during labor, and in the postpartum period.

Prepare the Nursery

Get the nursery ready, organize baby essentials, and ensure a welcoming environment for the newborn. Many new parents—mothers *and* fathers!—experience nesting during the last few weeks of pregnancy. They want to feel settled in their home and know they have everything ready for the baby. Most people think about the big-ticket items like a crib, changing table, dresser, stroller, and car seat. You might also want a comfortable recliner or rocking chair in the baby's room for feedings, bedtime stories, and cuddling them before naps. However, when it comes to supplies, you may also want to have a few boxes of diapers on hand in different sizes so you're never without them. Wipes are also a great item to stock up on since you know you'll be using them eventually. Instead of splurging on a lot of newborn clothes, buy clothes in multiple sizes. Get a few newborn outfits, but also several 0–3-month, 3–6-month, 6–9-month, and 9–12-month items. I usually tell new parents they can get away with a dozen onesies in each size because they're easy to put on and take off, and you can throw them in the wash. Trust me—you'll be doing a lot of laundry with a new baby! It's better to wash clothes often and re-wear them instead of having a whole drawer full of clothing the baby will never wear. They grow so quickly that you'll be surprised at how little time they stay in one size—and sometimes they completely skip a size during a growth spurt!

When it comes to doing your baby's laundry, use baby-safe laundry detergent to wash baby clothes, blankets, and linens. Avoid fabric softeners and harsh chemicals that may irritate the baby's sensitive skin. This may require some trial and error. I've had clients with fussy babies and they don't notice anything wrong—the baby is fed, dry, and just woke up from a nap. It's often a case of something in the detergent or fabric softener making the baby's skin feel itchy and uncomfortable.

Babies don't need many toys when they're young, but of course it's fun to buy stuffed animals, toys that have different textures, and cozy blankets to wrap them in. You can always put stuff like this on your baby registry. Whatever you get from a baby shower is good, but if you don't get everything, don't buy it immediately! You might find out that you don't need it at all, so you can save your time and money by waiting to see if your baby will need specific items.

Creating a safe and secure environment in your baby's nursery and crib is of utmost importance to ensure their well-being. Choose a crib that meets current safety standards. Look for certifications like ASTM International or Juvenile Products Manufacturers Association. Ensure the crib slats are no more than $2\frac{3}{8}$ inches apart to prevent the baby's head from getting stuck. Avoid using cribs with drop-side mechanisms, as they have been associated with safety hazards. Remove all soft bedding, including pillows, blankets, stuffed animals, and bumper pads, from the crib. These items can pose suffocation risks to infants less than a year old (M. Taylor, 2022). Use a firm mattress that fits the crib snugly with no more than two fingers' width between the mattress and the crib sides. Choose a mattress specifically designed for infants that meets all safety standards.

Put the baby to sleep on their back for all sleep times, including naps. Dress them in appropriate sleep clothing to prevent overheating, and avoid using heavy blankets or quilts. To ensure they get quality rest without getting too hot or cold, keep the room at a comfortable temperature to avoid extremes. Use a reliable baby monitor to keep an eye on your baby even when you're not in the room, but still regularly check on them when they're sleeping.

A changing table is a convenient and practical addition to your baby's nursery, but ensuring its safety is crucial to prevent accidents and injuries. As with any furniture in your house, secure it to the wall so it won't tip over. Some new parents use a dresser as a changing table due to the convenient drawers, so attach this to the wall and secure a changing pad to the top so it won't slip off when you're using it. If you're buying a new changing table, choose one that is sturdy, well-constructed, and designed specifically for changing diapers. Make sure it meets safety standards and has proper support. If your changing table has wheels, make sure they are locked before using the table. This prevents the table from moving while you're changing the baby.

Most changing tables and pads come with a safety strap that helps secure the baby in place during diaper changes. Always use this strap, even if you believe your baby can't roll over yet. They can wiggle their way around even when they're little, and your grip may not be enough to hold them in place while you're grabbing supplies.

With that in mind, organize diapers, wipes, creams, and other essentials within arm's reach before placing the baby on the changing table. This prevents you from needing to turn away to retrieve items during the diaper change. Never leave your baby unattended on the changing table, even for a moment. Babies can roll unexpectedly, and falls from even a short height can cause serious injuries. While changing the baby, always keep one hand on them. This provides an added layer of security in case they attempt to roll or move.

Place a changing pad or mat on top of the changing table to create a comfortable and soft surface for the baby. This can also help prevent them from sliding. Keep the changing area clutter-free to prevent accidentally knocking items off the table or causing distractions during diaper changes. Avoid hanging heavy items or decorations directly above the changing table. This reduces the risk of items falling onto the baby during a diaper change. If you're disposing of soiled diapers in a trash bin located near the changing table, ensure it has a secure lid to prevent curious hands from reaching in.

Diaper changes can sometimes be a bit challenging, especially with a fidgety baby. Stay calm, focused, and patient to avoid any accidental mishaps. Always prioritize your baby's safety during diaper changes and maintain constant supervision to prevent any accidents.

Babyproof the House

We addressed babyproofing in Chapter 4, so refer back to that section to ensure you cover all your bases with babyproofing before you bring home your baby. This is essential to their safety once they start moving independently, but it's better to do it all before the baby's born to ensure you have the time and energy to do it properly. At the very least, you need to install safety gates at the top and bottom of stairs, cover electrical outlets, secure furniture and heavy objects to walls, and use corner guards on sharp edges.

Babyproof the kitchen by securing cabinets and drawers, and ensure hazardous items like cleaning products are out of reach. In the bathroom, use nonslip mats and keep medicines and toiletries in a secure place.

Babyproofing doesn't only refer to safety issues! You might want to consider the noise levels of your home, too. I've had many clients invest in white noise machines for the baby's room. These devices make calming noises to soothe the baby to sleep. It also prevents them from being in total silence, which makes it less likely that they'll wake up if someone rings the doorbell or you and your wife try to watch a movie after they've gone to bed!

Get Ready for Labor

Pack a hospital bag with essentials for your stay during the birth, including comfortable clothes and toiletries for your wife, plus items for the baby.

As the due date draws closer, you may want to join parenting forums or support groups to connect with other expectant parents and share experiences. You can meet these parents in your prenatal classes or online forums. You can also use this time to have open discussions with your partner about parenting roles and responsibilities to ensure you are on the same page.

Labor

Preparing for labor is essential to help ensure a smooth and comfortable birthing experience. While labor can be unpredictable, having an action plan in place can provide guidance and support during this transformative time. As your partner goes into labor, make sure you grab the hospital bag and your wallet, keys, phone, and other necessary items. Don't put it on her to remember to take anything, because she may already be consumed by contractions and discomfort! Once you're at the hospital or birthing center, you can use these tips to ensure things go as smoothly as possible.

Manage Your Emotions

Labor can be intense, but staying calm and focused can help manage anxiety and stress. Remember that however anxious you feel, your partner is experiencing that exponentially! While you want to remain calm so she knows she can depend on you, try to put her first whenever possible.

Support Your Partner

Practice deep breathing and relaxation techniques with your partner so she can stay centered during contractions. Position changes can also help her manage pain and discomfort during labor. Help her utilize comfort measures to cope with contractions and pain. This may include walking, rocking, massage, warm compresses, or taking a warm bath or shower—all of which you can assist with!

Ensure she drinks fluids and consumes light snacks if her health-care provider allows it. Staying hydrated and nourished can help maintain her energy levels during labor.

Your partner should feel encouraged to advocate for herself, but if she's unable to or isn't being heard, you need to step up for her. Share preferences or concerns by communicating clearly with the health-care provider. Both you and your partner have the right to be active participants in the birthing process.

Communicate Openly

Effective communication with health-care providers can help you understand what's happening and make informed decisions. Check in with your partner often to ensure she's feeling supported and knows how much progress she's made. Having a supportive partner or birth coach can provide emotional and physical assistance during labor. Even if you and your partner hired a doula, make sure you're there, too, so your partner doesn't feel abandoned.

Consider Pain Management

Discuss pain relief options with your partner's health-care provider in advance. This may include nonmedical techniques like breathing techniques or medical interventions such as epidurals. Be open to adjusting your birth plan based on your needs.

Stay Flexible

Labor can be unpredictable; be open to changes in the birth plan based on the health and well-being of both the baby and the mother. However, you should also trust your instincts. Your partner's body will know what to do during labor, so make sure you check in with her and make her needs heard to the medical professionals. Take care of everything you can to help so your partner only needs to focus on giving birth.

It can also be a lengthy process. Stay positive and patient, knowing that each contraction brings you closer to meeting your baby. Never falter in being available for your partner. Stay by her side throughout labor and be actively engaged in the process. Your presence and support can make a significant difference to her emotional well-being.

If your partner is comfortable with it, take photos or videos to capture the special moments of labor and the baby's first moments after birth. Even though she's the one experiencing it, she most likely won't remember it after the fact—many women run on adrenaline and fumes during labor. She also isn't able to see things from the same angle as you, so you can capture sweet shots with her holding the baby for the first time.

Keep in mind that the ultimate goal is to welcome a healthy baby into the world. Stay positive and focused on the joyous outcome. By being a caring and supportive presence during labor, new dads can create a positive and empowering birthing experience for their partner, setting the foundation for a strong bond between the family members as they welcome their new addition to the world.

Postpartum

Planning for the postpartum period is essential because it's a significant and transformative time for both the new mother and the entire family. Postpartum is the period immediately after childbirth and typically lasts for about six weeks, but planning for the entire fourth trimester can ensure you, your partner, and your new baby have all the support you need to adjust to this new phase of life.

Prioritize Your Partner

Welcoming a new baby can impact the dynamics of a relationship. Planning for postpartum includes open communication with partners about expectations and roles during this time. You and your wife can talk about your parenting goals and roles before you bring home the baby to ensure a smooth transition. It will also help you know how you can support her while she heals and bonds with the baby in the first few weeks postpartum.

The mother's body undergoes significant changes during pregnancy and childbirth. Planning for postpartum allows the mother to focus on her physical recovery, ensuring she gets the rest, nutrition, and medical care needed to heal properly. Allow ample time for postpartum recovery so your partner doesn't feel pressured to do more than her body can handle.

Postpartum emotions can be intense and varied, ranging from joy and excitement to feelings of overwhelm and sadness. Planning ahead can help address emotional challenges and provide support for the new mother's mental health. Still, even if you're prepared, you should be aware of the signs of PPD and seek professional help if you or your partner experience persistent feelings of sadness, anxiety, or difficulty coping.

Being prepared for adjusting at home with the baby allows you to address any potential postpartum health concerns promptly. It ensures that the mother receives the necessary medical attention and monitoring during her recovery.

For mothers who plan to breastfeed, postpartum planning involves learning about breastfeeding, setting up a comfortable nursing space, and seeking professional support if needed. You can learn along with your partner and ensure you always give her time and space to breastfeed.

Ways to support your partner during that time include giving her snacks and water so she can keep her supply up and not get dehydrated while she feeds the baby. You can also take care of practical matters like washing the pump parts. Familiarize yourself with the pump and its components. Understand the manufacturer's guidelines for cleaning and sterilizing the parts. After each pumping session, disassemble the pump and wash the parts promptly to prevent the milk residue from drying. Wash the parts with warm, soapy water using a mild dish soap that is safe for cleaning baby-related items. Make sure to clean all parts thoroughly, including valves, membranes, and connectors. After washing, rinse all the parts thoroughly with clean water to ensure there is no soap residue left behind. Allow the pump parts to air dry on a clean surface or use a clean towel to dry them. Avoid using paper towels, as they can leave fibers on the parts. Once the pump parts are completely dry, store them in a clean, dry container or a designated area until they're needed again. Keep the pump charged so it's ready when your partner needs it. You can track her breastfeeding schedule and charge the pump each time, let it charge overnight, or check the battery levels a bit before she'll need to use it. These seemingly small tasks can make a significant difference in a breastfeeding mom's experience, allowing her to focus more on nurturing her baby and herself.

Bond With Your Baby

Spend quality time bonding with the baby through skin-to-skin contact, talking, singing, and gentle touch. Bonding can help in building a strong parent–child relationship. But remember that caring for a newborn can be demanding and exhausting. Planning for postpartum allows you and your partner to make arrangements for sharing responsibilities and ensuring the baby's needs are met. You want to share the workload to ensure you're both caring for and bonding with your baby while also getting time to rest and enjoy your hobbies or downtime.

Take Care of Yourself

Having a postpartum plan in place can significantly reduce stress and overwhelm during the early weeks after childbirth. It provides a roadmap for you to navigate this life-changing period more smoothly. So as you plan for life with a new baby, ensure you make time for yourself.

Newborns have irregular sleep patterns, and sleep deprivation is common for parents. Planning for postpartum can involve finding ways to ensure both parents get sufficient rest to cope with the demands of caring for a newborn.

Prioritize self-care by engaging in activities you enjoy, seeking emotional support from your partner or support network, and considering postpartum exercises or relaxation techniques to reduce stress.

Accept Help

Planning ahead allows the new parents to identify their support network, including family, friends, or professionals who can provide emotional support and guidance during this transitional period.

Don't hesitate to accept help from family and friends. Let them assist with household chores, cooking, or taking care of the baby, allowing you to rest and recover.

Postpartum Support Checklist for New Dads

After childbirth, new dads play a crucial role in supporting both the new mother and the baby during the postpartum period. These actionable tips will help new dads navigate the early days after childbirth:

- **Provide emotional support.** Be emotionally present and supportive for the new mother. Offer words of encouragement and reassurance, as she may experience a range of emotions during this time. Always be available to listen to her and make her feel heard and supported.

- **Help with household chores.** Take on household chores and responsibilities to allow the new mother to focus on rest and recovery. This can include cooking, cleaning, laundry, and grocery shopping. Remember to outsource these tasks if possible to prevent overextending yourself when you need to help your partner.

- **Assist with baby care.** Be actively involved in caring for the baby. Help with diaper changes, bathing, and soothing the baby when needed. Support your wife while she breastfeeds and offer to help with bottle-feeding, whether it's pumped milk or formula. When your wife breastfeeds, you can help by positioning and burping the baby, and bringing snacks or water to the nursing area.

- **Encourage rest and sleep.** Encourage the new mother to rest and get sufficient sleep. Take turns caring for the baby during the night to ensure both parents get enough rest. Shifts are ideal for this, but you'll find what works best for you and your partner. While you want to ensure she gets plenty of rest, you also need to get sleep so you can be a helpful and supportive partner.

- **Facilitate bonding time.** Encourage bonding time between the new mother and the baby. Support skin-to-skin contact, and encourage breastfeeding if applicable. You can also bond with the baby using skin-to-skin contact. Talk to your baby during this time, or read to them and sing lullabies to them so they'll learn your voice.

- **Be patient and understanding.** Understand that the postpartum period can be challenging for both the new mother and the baby. Be patient and offer understanding during this adjustment period. Don't react from a place of hurt or anger; give yourself time to process what was said or done and calm down before you speak or react harshly. Tempers are short or nonexistent during this period, so don't let it get the best of you both.

- **Communicate openly.** Have open and honest communication with your partner. Discuss any concerns or challenges and work together as a team to find solutions. Again, wait to react to things until you have time to process what was said and can think through your response. But that doesn't mean you should hold back. Always say what you think so there's no resentment building in your relationship.

- **Monitor postpartum health.** Keep an eye on the new mother's physical and emotional well-being. If any concerns arise, encourage her to seek medical or professional support. Some new mothers may notice they're acting in a different way or feel depressed long past the baby blues stage, but you should also be aware of the signs as discussed in Chapter 3. If you're also supporting your partner and looking out for her mental health, she'll have the best chance at early detection and prompt treatment of any issues in her postpartum period.

- **Attend medical appointments.** Accompany the new mother and baby to doctor's appointments. Be actively involved in understanding the baby's health and development. You want to be there so you're informed about the baby's health but also to support your wife, so she isn't taking a newborn to doctor's appointments alone during her postpartum healing.

- **Plan special moments.** Plan special moments for your new family, such as taking family photos, going for a walk together, or having a simple celebration at home. Take photos and document the baby's milestones; it's a great way to cherish and preserve precious memories. You might feel like this is going above and beyond—and it is! But don't think it's something you should also just let fall to the wayside while you adjust to your growing family. These events will be so special to your wife and make her feel appreciated. My new mom clients always say that they take the photos but are never in them, so be sure to capture some sweet moments between your wife and her new baby during this time!

- **Encourage self-care.** Encourage the new mother to practice self-care and take time for herself. Offer to take care of the baby while she engages in activities she enjoys. Of course, as I've stated throughout this book, your self-care is also crucial! But as a partner, you should put the new mother ahead of yourself. She's healing physically and emotionally, so you're starting off in a better position than her. Yes, you'll both experience diaper blowouts and sleepless nights, but if she feels like you're encouraging her self-care, she'll turn around and do the same for you, which will make your relationship even stronger in the process.

- **Seek support together.** Attend postpartum support groups or classes together, where both parents can learn about infant care and parenting and connect with other new parents. Hopefully my stories at the beginning of each chapter have helped you realize that it's always best to ask for help! You don't have to hire a one-on-one professional like me, but support groups and parenting classes can greatly help you feel more supported as new parents. You might think you already know everything you need to become a great dad, but these classes might help you find new ways to approach things, like parenting hacks to streamline the process! If nothing else, you and your wife will be on the same page regarding this type of parenting information and may even make some new parent friends.

- **Share your feelings.** Share your own feelings and experiences as a new dad. It's essential to communicate and support each other through this new journey. You want to ensure your wife speaks out and is heard first, as she went through a painful physical experience to become a mother, but you don't need to bite your tongue. You're an equal partner in this family, so speak up and make sure she knows you're just as invested as she is.

- **Be involved in decision-making.** Part of speaking up and sharing your feelings is staying involved. Be actively involved in making decisions about parenting, routines, and other aspects of caring for the baby. While you might think your wife is more invested since she carried and gave birth to the baby, you should establish yourself as an equal partner. If you step back and let your wife take the lead, you might miss out on key times to bond with your baby and ensure you're an active parent in their life. Remember, decision-making is just as much about your baby as it is the parents. You should strive to provide the best for your child.

- **Be flexible and adapt.** Recognize that parenthood is a learning process. Be flexible and adapt to the needs of the baby and the family as they evolve. Thinking everything will play out one way can mean you're easily thrown off course if something doesn't go according to plan. It's ideal to have action plans in place, especially with tips like these that can apply at any time, anywhere. But you should also feel prepared to change plans at the drop of a hat. If you don't learn this before bringing your baby home, you'll definitely learn it the first time they blow out a diaper in public, then spit up all over the backup outfit and have you racing home to get everyone clean!

Dads have a unique and essential role in the early stages of a baby's life. By being actively involved, supportive, and present, dads can strengthen their bond with the baby and support the new mother during the postpartum period. This active engagement will contribute to the overall well-being and happiness of the entire family. But remember, every experience is unique. The most important thing is to be present, supportive, and loving as you embark on this new journey together. Celebrate the joys and work through the challenges as a team, and you will help create a strong and loving foundation for your new family.

By following a personalized action plan, new parents can better prepare themselves for the challenges of childbirth and postpartum, enabling them to embrace this transformative journey with more confidence and resilience. Remember that seeking professional guidance and support when needed is crucial, and there is no shame in asking for help during this significant life transition.

In Our Session

If we were having a one-on-one session about developing or implementing your action plan during pregnancy, labor, and postpartum, I would ask about your perceived level of preparedness, your support system, and your flexibility:

- What are your expectations for fatherhood? How do you envision your role as a dad?

- What are you most looking forward to in becoming a father?

- How prepared do you feel for the responsibilities and challenges that come with fatherhood?

- Are there specific aspects of fatherhood that you feel confident about? Are there areas where you feel less prepared?

- What steps have you taken to educate yourself about pregnancy, childbirth, and parenting? Have you attended any classes or workshops?

- Are there any specific areas of parenting that you're interested in learning more about?

- Have you and your partner sought support from external sources, such as friends, family, or counseling, to navigate these relationship changes? How open are you to seeking support if needed?

- How have you personally grown and adapted as a partner and as a parent since the baby's arrival?

- In what ways have you witnessed positive changes in your relationship despite the challenges that come with parenthood?

Conclusion

In the journey of becoming new parents, the postpartum period, often referred to as the fourth trimester, is a crucial phase that demands the utmost attention, care, and understanding. I wrote *The Postpartum Book for Partners* with the intention of providing a comprehensive and insightful guide to support partners during this transformative time. We have explored the physical, emotional, and psychological challenges that arise after childbirth, emphasizing the significance of self-care while supporting a new mother.

However, throughout this book, we have stressed the importance of recognizing that the postpartum experience is not solely about the new mother; it's a shared journey between partners. Balancing the roles of a supportive partner and a new parent can be challenging, but with the right knowledge, empathy, and communication it becomes a deeply fulfilling experience for both partners.

Becoming a father is a momentous occasion, and it comes with its own set of challenges and joys. Throughout this book, we have emphasized the importance of active involvement, communication, and empathy in your new role. Understanding the physical and emotional changes that your wife is going through postpartum is key to providing the support and care she needs.

Understanding the physical changes and hormonal fluctuations that new mothers undergo is crucial for partners to provide the needed support and reassurance. By acknowledging the emotional roller coaster that many new mothers experience, partners can create an environment of understanding and comfort. Offering a listening ear and a shoulder to lean on, and validating her emotions, goes a long way in helping new mothers navigate the challenges of the postpartum period.

As a new dad, you should recognize that your partnership with your wife extends beyond sharing responsibilities; it also involves emotional support and being a reliable pillar during moments of vulnerability. Be present, listen with an open heart, and offer reassurance during the highs and lows of new parenthood.

You've learned practical tips, from assisting with baby care tasks to maintaining a healthy balance between work, family, and personal time. Embracing teamwork in parenting ensures that both partners feel valued and supported, fostering a strong and nurturing environment for your baby's growth and development.

In addition to stressing the need to support the new mother, this book has highlighted the significance of not neglecting yourself in the process. Partners must remember that they, too, are experiencing a transition to parenthood, which can be equally overwhelming and transformative. Finding time for self-care, seeking support from friends and family, and openly communicating feelings and concerns are vital steps in maintaining a strong and healthy partnership during the postpartum period.

We've also recognized the importance of teamwork and the power of sharing responsibilities in parenting. Equitable distribution of tasks, from feeding and diaper changes to household chores, fosters a sense of partnership and alleviates the burden on both parents. This not only strengthens the bond between partners but also allows the new mother to focus on her recovery and bonding with the baby.

While I can't help each of you one on one as I do many clients, I want you to get one main idea from this book, even if you take away nothing else. *The Postpartum Book for Partners* stresses the need to foster open conversations about postpartum mental health and the potential challenges that arise. Recognizing the signs of PPD and postpartum anxiety is essential for partners to support their loved ones and seek professional help when necessary. Remember, it's okay to ask for assistance and seek guidance in navigating this delicate phase—for both you and the new mother.

You should approach the postpartum period with compassion, patience, and love. Embrace the beauty of this transformative time and cherish the moments of growth, joy, and connection that come with it instead of focusing on the stress and sleep deprivation. By working together and prioritizing the well-being of both partners, the journey into parenthood can become an enriching and rewarding experience.

Above all, remember that every family's postpartum experience is unique. I worked to establish this in the opening case studies of each chapter, which show different sides to the same situation. I want to show that there is no one-size-fits-all approach to childbirth, the postpartum period, and partner support. Be flexible, be kind to yourselves, and trust in your love and commitment to one another. With the knowledge gained from this book and an unwavering dedication to the partnership, you will not only navigate the fourth trimester but also lay the foundation for a lifetime of love, trust, and happiness in your new role as parents.

References

Adjusting to early parenthood. (2023, March 28). COPE. https://www.cope.org.au/new-parents/first-weeks/

Adjusting to parenthood. (2020, May 28). Beyond Blue. https://healthyfamilies.beyondblue.org.au/pregnancy-and-new-parents/becoming-a-parent-what-to-expect/adjusting-to-parenthood

Bell, S. (2021, September). *Seven steps to creating a successful baby routine.* BabyCentre. https://www.babycentre.co.uk/a1051918/seven-steps-to-creating-a-successful-baby-routine

Bernard-Bonnin, A.-C. (2006). Feeding problems of infants and toddlers. *Canadian Family Physician, 52*(10), 1247–1251. https://www.ncbi.nlm.nih.gov/pmc/articles/PMC1783606/

Bouffard, S. (2020, March 17). *How to make a new home routine.* PBS Kids for Parents. https://www.pbs.org/parents/thrive/schools-closed-how-to-make-a-new-home-routine

Bykofsky, M. (2023, June 27). *6 steps to babyproofing your house: A checklist for every room.* Parents. https://www.parents.com/baby/safety/babyproofing/babyproofing-your-home-from-top-to-bottom/

Chauhan, G., & Tadi, P. (2020). *Physiology, postpartum changes.* StatPearls Publishing. https://www.ncbi.nlm.nih.gov/books/NBK555904/

Chuck, E., & McShane, J. (2023, January 30). *What is postpartum psychosis? Rare condition is in the spotlight after the killing of three children in Massachusetts.* NBC News. https://www.nbcnews.com/news/us-news/postpartum-psychosis-rare-condition-spotlight-killing-three-children-m-rcna68165

Coleman, P. A. (2022, July 28). *New dad survival tips to get you through the first month*. Fatherly. https://www.fatherly.com/parenting/new-dad-survival-tips-first-month

Collier, S. (2021, July 30). *Postpartum anxiety is invisible, but common and treatable*. Harvard Health Publishing. https://www.health.harvard.edu/blog/postpartum-anxiety-an-invisible-disorder-that-can-affect-new-mothers-202107302558

Coping with the neonatal intensive care unit (NICU): Tips. (n.d.). Raising Children Network. https://raisingchildren.net.au/newborns/premature-babies-sick-babies/neonatal-intensive-care/coping-with-nicu

Curtis-Mahoney, C., & Reilly, N. (2022, August 3). *Top tips for new parents*. William James College. https://www.williamjames.edu/centers-and-services/forensic-and-clinical-services/yfps/tips-for-parents/top-ten-tips-new-parents.html

de Aguiar, A. S. C., Ximenes, L. B., Lúcio, I. M. L., Pagliuca, L. M. F., & Cardoso, M. V. L. M. L. (2011). Association of the red reflex in newborns with neonatal variables. *Revista Latino-Americana de Enfermagem, 19*(2), 309–316. https://doi.org/10.1590/S0104-11692011000200012

de Bellefonds, C. (2022, April 26). *How soon after giving birth can you get pregnant?* What to Expect. https://www.whattoexpect.com/pregnancy/pregnancy-health/how-soon-can-you-get-pregnant-after-giving-birth/

Dennis, C.-L., Brown, H. K., & Brennenstuhl, S. (2017). The Postpartum Partner Support Scale: Development, psychometric assessment, and predictive validity in a Canadian prospective cohort. *Midwifery, 54,* 18–24. https://doi.org/10.1016/j.midw.2017.07.018

Depression in pregnancy. (2021, November 9). National Health Service. https://www.nhs.uk/pregnancy/keeping-well/depression/

Desai, N. M., & Tsukerman, A. (2021). *Vaginal delivery.* StatPearls Publishing. https://www.ncbi.nlm.nih.gov/books/NBK559197/

Diamond, R. (2023, March 10). *Communication and intimacy tools for new parents.* Psychology Today. https://www.psychologytoday.com/us/blog/preparing-for-parenthood/202303/communication-and-intimacy-tools-for-new-parents

Divecha, D. (2016, May 4). *Ten changes new parents face.* Greater Good. https://greatergood.berkeley.edu/article/item/ten_changes_new_parents_face

Dougherty, E. (2022, July 28). *Baby schedules: Why, when, and how to start a daily routine with your baby.* BabyCenter. https://www.babycenter.com/baby/schedules/the-basics-of-baby-schedules-why-when-and-how-to-start-a-rou_3658352

Eldemire, A. (2021, April 29). *The one conversation that new parents need to stay connected.* The Gottman Institute. https://www.gottman.com/blog/one-conversation-new-parents-need-stay-connected/

EmpathicParentingCounseling. *Establishing routines with a newborn: Tips for parents.* (2023, July 27). Empathetic Parenting Counselinghttps://empathicparentingcounseling.com/blog/establishing-routines-with-a-newborn

First-time dad tips—how to be a hands-on dad. (n.d.). SMA Nutrition. https://www.smababy.co.uk/pregnancy/tips-on-being-a-first-time-dad

Fischer, K. (2022, January 25). *How to tell if your child has a feeding problem—and what to do next.* Motherly. https://www.mother.ly/baby/baby-feeding-guides-schedules/spotting-feeding-problems-in-children/

Fletcher, C. (2023, March 8). *How new parents can create – and maintain – a morning routine.* ParentCo. https://www.parent.com/blogs/conversations/how-new-parents-can-create-and-maintain-a-morning-routine

Fletcher, J. (2022, August 12). *Relationships after having a baby: What to expect and how to cope.* Psych Central. https://psychcentral.com/relationships/tips-to-help-reconnect-with-your-partner-after-baby

Fletcher, J., & Craft, C. (2022, August 30). *How parenting during the infant and toddler years can affect child development.* Psych Central. https://psychcentral.com/health/purposeful-parenting-the-infant-or-toddler

Geddes, J. K. (2021, April 26). *Postpartum obsessive-compulsive disorder (OCD).* What to Expect. https://www.whattoexpect.com/first-year/postpartum-health-and-care/postpartum-obsessive-compulsive-disorder

Geddes, J. K. (2022, August 12). *How to babyproof every room of the house.* What to Expect. https://www.whattoexpect.com/nursery-decorating/childproofing-basics.aspx

Gorbis, E. (2023, May 2). *Understanding postpartum OCD and the mother/baby attachment.* Anxiety and Depression Association of America. https://adaa.org/learn-from-us/from-the-experts/blog-posts/consumer/unexpected-ocd-postpartum

Horsager-Boehrer, R. (2021, August 17). *1 in 10 dads experience postpartum depression, anxiety: How to spot the signs.* UT Southwestern Medical Center. https://utswmed.org/medblog/paternal-postpartum-depression/

How to create a daily routine for new moms. (2021, January 25). Making Time for Giggles. https://makingtimeforgiggles.com/daily-routines-for-new-moms/

Hudak, R., & Wisner, K. L. (2012). Diagnosis and treatment of postpartum obsessions and compulsions that involve infant harm. *American Journal of Psychiatry*, *169*(4), 360–363. https://doi.org/10.1176/appi.ajp.2011.11050667

Jondle, J. (2019, August 29). *What you need to know about postpartum anxiety.* Healthline. https://www.healthline.com/health/pregnancy/postpartum-anxiety

Jones, I., Cantwell, R., & on behalf of the Nosology Working Group, Royal College of Psychiatrists, Perinatal Section. (2010). The classification of perinatal mood disorders—suggestions for DSMV and ICD11. *Archives of Women's Mental Health*, *13*(1), 33–36. https://doi.org/10.1007/s00737-009-0122-1

Jullien, S. (2021). Vision screening in newborns and early childhood. *BMC Pediatrics*, *21*, 306. https://doi.org/10.1186/s12887-021-02606-2

Karp, H. (n.d.). *Advice for new parents: 9 tips from Dr. Harvey Karp.* Happiest Baby. https://www.happiestbaby.com/blogs/parents/new-parent-tips

Kerr, M. (2023, March 23). *Perinatal depression.* Healthline. https://www.healthline.com/health/depression/perinatal-depression

Klass, P., & Damour, L. (2019). How to be a modern parent. *The New York Times.* https://www.nytimes.com/guides/well/guide-to-modern-parenting

Lambert, K. (2009, March 11). *5 things to know about adjusting to parenthood.* HowStuffWorks. https://lifestyle.howstuffworks.com/family/parenting/parenting-tips/5-things-to-know-about-adjusting-to-parenthood.htm

Letko, J. (2019, October 28). *Kegels: The 30-second exercise that can improve incontinence and sex.* UChicago Medicine.

https://www.uchicagomedicine.org/forefront/womens-health-articles/kegels-the-30-second-exercise-that-can-improve-incontinence-and-sex

Li, X. F., Fortney, J. A., Kotelchuck, M., & Glover, L. H. (1996). The postpartum period: The key to maternal mortality. *International Journal of Gynecology & Obstetrics, 54*(1), 1–10. https://doi.org/10.1016/0020-7292(96)02667-7

Martin, J. A., Hamilton, B. E., Osterman, M. J. K., Driscoll, A. K., & Mathews, T. J. (2017). Births: Final data for 2015. *National Vital Statistics Reports, 66*(1). https://www.cdc.gov/nchs/data/nvsr/nvsr66/nvsr66_01.pdf

Mayo Clinic Staff. (2022, January 25). *Depression during pregnancy: You're not alone.* Mayo Clinic. https://www.mayoclinic.org/healthy-lifestyle/pregnancy-week-by-week/in-depth/depression-during-pregnancy/art-20237875

McCallum, K. (2021, February 17). *Postpartum exercise: What to know about exercising after pregnancy.* Houston Methodist. https://www.houstonmethodist.org/blog/articles/2021/feb/postpartum-exercise-what-to-know-about-exercising-after-pregnancy/

Miller, E. S., Chu, C., Gollan, J., & Gossett, D. R. (2013). Obsessive-compulsive symptoms during the postpartum period. *The Journal of Reproductive Medicine, 58*(3–4), 115–122. https://www.ncbi.nlm.nih.gov/pmc/articles/PMC5705036/

Mishra, S., Agarwal, R., Deorari, A. K., & Paul, V. K. (2008). Jaundice in the newborns. *The Indian Journal of Pediatrics, 75*(2), 157–163. https://doi.org/10.1007/s12098-008-0024-7

Nakić Radoš, S., Tadinac, M., & Herman, R. (2018). Anxiety during pregnancy and postpartum: Course, predictors and comorbidity with postpartum depression. *Acta Clinica Croatica, 57*(1), 39–51. https://doi.org/10.20471/acc.2018.57.01.05

Nathanson, A. (2019, January 11). *Post-baby communication problems? 7 ways to reconnect.* Zencare. https://blog.zencare.co/communication-problems-new-parents/

National Institute of Mental Health. (2021). *Perinatal depression.* https://www.nimh.nih.gov/health/publications/perinatal-depression

Neonatal intensive care unit (NICU): Common problems. (2017, October 17). Pampers. https://www.pampers.com/en-us/baby/newborn/article/common-nicu-conditions-and-treatments

Neu, J., & Rushing, J. (2011). Cesarean versus vaginal delivery: Long-term infant outcomes and the hygiene hypothesis. *Clinics in Perinatology, 38*(2), 321–331. https://doi.org/10.1016/j.clp.2011.03.008

Newborn hearing screening. (2020, May 26). Centers for Disease Control and Prevention. https://www.cdc.gov/ncbddd/hearingloss/parentsguide/understanding/newbornhearingscreening.html

Newman, T. B., Easterling, M. J., Goldman, E. S., & Stevenson, D. K. (1990). Laboratory evaluation of jaundice in newborns. *American Journal of Diseases of Children, 144*(3), 364. https://doi.org/10.1001/archpedi.1990.02150270114039

Novak, S. (2022, January 19). *What to do and how to cope when your preemie's in the NICU.* What to Expect. https://www.whattoexpect.com/first-year/baby-care/how-parents-can-cope-when-premature-baby-is-in-nicu/

Perinatal mood and anxiety disorders. (n.d.). Center for Women's Mood Disorders. https://www.med.unc.edu/psych/wmd/resources/mood-disorders/perinatal/

Perinatal or postpartum mood and anxiety disorders. (2018, October 19). The Children's Hospital of Philadelphia. https://www.chop.edu/conditions-diseases/perinatal-or-postpartum-mood-and-anxiety-disorders

Pietrangelo, A. (2022, March 31). *Everything you need to know about postpartum depression: Symptoms, treatments, and finding help.* Healthline. https://www.healthline.com/health/depression/postpartum-depression

Postpartum post-traumatic stress disorder. (2014). Postpartum Support International. https://www.postpartum.net/learn-more/postpartum-post-traumatic-stress-disorder/

Postpartum psychosis. (2014). Postpartum Support International. https://www.postpartum.net/learn-more/postpartum-psychosis/

Raza, S. K., & Raza, S. (2022). *Postpartum psychosis.* StatPearls Publishing. https://www.ncbi.nlm.nih.gov/books/NBK544304/

Ringley, T. (2021, July 29). *10 things your NICU nurses wish you knew.* Verywell Family. https://www.verywellfamily.com/things-nicu-nurses-wish-you-knew-2748402

Rodriguez, A. (2019, November 26). *How to tell if your baby has a feeding problem.* Edward-Elmhurst Health. https://www.eehealth.org/blog/2019/11/feeding-disorder/

Romano, M., Cacciatore, A., Giordano, R., & La Rosa, B. (2010). Postpartum period: Three distinct but continuous phases. *Journal of Prenatal Medicine, 4*(2), 22–25. https://www.ncbi.nlm.nih.gov/pmc/articles/PMC3279173/

Ross, L. E., Murray, B. J., & Steiner, M. (2005). Sleep and perinatal mood disorders: A critical review. *Journal of Psychiatry & Neuroscience, 30*(4), 247–256. https://www.ncbi.nlm.nih.gov/pmc/articles/PMC1160560/

Salazar, S. (2019, July 4). *How to adapt your lifestyle when you become a parent.* Our Family Lifestyle. https://ourfamilylifestyle.com/how-to-adapt-your-lifestyle-when-you-become-a-parent/

Sayad, E., & Silva-Carmona, M. (2020). *Meconium aspiration.* StatPearls Publishing. https://www.ncbi.nlm.nih.gov/books/NBK557425/

Schwab, W., Marth, C., & Bergant, A. (2012). Post-traumatic stress disorder post partum. *Geburtshilfe Und Frauenheilkunde, 72*(01), 56–63. https://doi.org/10.1055/s-0031-1280408

Shatzman, C. (2023, January 31). *15 plants found in or around your home that are poisonous for sids.* The Bump. https://www.thebump.com/a/poisonous-plants-for-kids

Shields, S. G., Ratcliffe, S. D., Fontaine, P., & Leeman, L. (2007). Dystocia in nulliparous women. *American Family Physician, 75*(11), 1671–1678. https://www.aafp.org/pubs/afp/issues/2007/0601/p1671.html

Slack, G. (2021, July 21). *10 tips for new dads.* WebMD. https://www.webmd.com/parenting/baby/ten-suggestions-for-new-dads

Slivinski, N. (2022, December 9). *Postpartum psychosis: What it is and what to do about it.* WebMD. https://www.webmd.com/parenting/baby/postpartum-psychosis-overview

Stranges, E., Wier, L., & Elixhauser, A. (2012). *Complicating conditions of vaginal deliveries and cesarean sections, 2009.* Agency for Healthcare Research and Quality. https://hcup-us.ahrq.gov/reports/statbriefs/sb131.pdf

Taylor, M. (2022, July 15). *Crib safety.* What to Expect. https://www.whattoexpect.com/pregnancy/ask-heidi/crib-safety.aspx

Taylor, N. (2022, February 28). *Tips for new dads: 33 tips that are great advice for expectant fathers and first time dads.* Fathercraft. https://fathercraft.com/new-dad-tips/

Taylor, R. B. (2008, October 28). *Breastfeeding overview.* WebMD; WebMD. https://www.webmd.com/parenting/baby/nursing-basics

Uludağ, E., & Öztürk, S. (2020). The effect of partner support on self-efficiency in breastfeeding in the early postpartum period. *The American Journal of Family Therapy, 48*(2), 211–219. https://doi.org/10.1080/01926187.2019.1697973

Watson, K. (2020, October 6). *Life after delivery.* Healthline. https://www.healthline.com/health/pregnancy/life-after-delivery

Waychoff, A. (2020, October 12). *A guide on effective couple-based communication after baby.* Hello Postpartum. https://hellopostpartum.com/couple-communication-tips-baby/

When your baby's in the NICU (for parents). (2019, January). Nemours KidsHealth. https://kidshealth.org/en/parents/nicu-caring.html

Wisner, W. (2022, July 25). *What is prenatal or perinatal depression?* Verywell Family. https://www.verywellfamily.com/prenatal-depression-4846439

Wroblewska-Seniuk, K. E., Dabrowski, P., Szyfter, W., & Mazela, J. (2016). Universal newborn hearing screening: Methods and results, obstacles, and benefits. *Pediatric Research, 81*(3), 415–422. https://doi.org/10.1038/pr.2016.250

Your baby's hearing screening and next steps. (2021, October). National Institute on Deafness and Other Communication Disorders. https://www.nidcd.nih.gov/health/your-babys-hearing-screening-and-next-steps

Your body after baby: The first 6 weeks. (2018, July). March of Dimes. https://www.marchofdimes.org/find-support/topics/postpartum/your-body-after-baby-first-6-weeks

Made in the USA
Columbia, SC
10 May 2024

35533665R00088